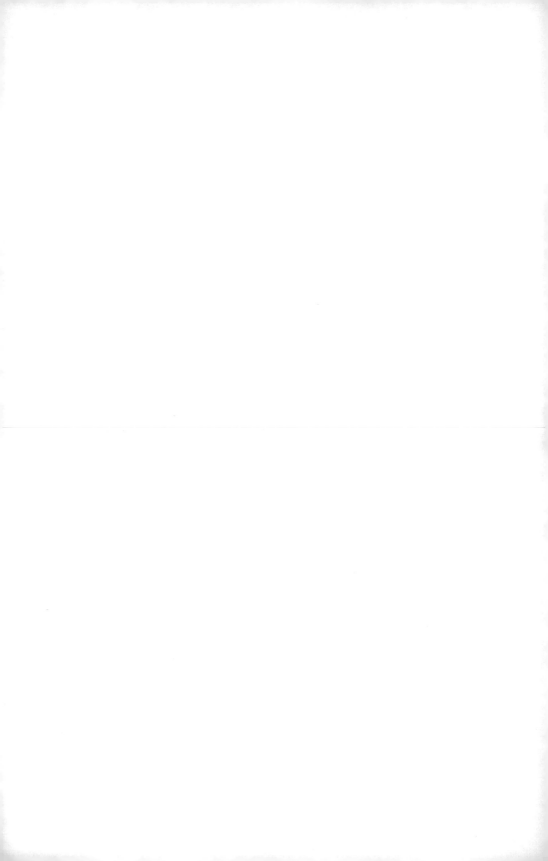

Plague Years

Ross A. Slotten, MD

Plague

A DOCTOR'S JOURNEY THROUGH

Years

THE AIDS CRISIS

THE UNIVERSITY OF CHICAGO PRESS

Chicago and London

The University of Chicago Press, Chicago 60637
The University of Chicago Press, Ltd., London
© 2020 by The University of Chicago
All rights reserved. No part of this book may be used or reproduced
in any manner whatsoever without written permission, except in the case
of brief quotations in critical articles and reviews. For more information,
contact the University of Chicago Press, 1427 E. 60th St., Chicago, IL 60637.
Published 2020
Printed in the United States of America

29 28 27 26 25 24 23 22 21 20   1 2 3 4 5

ISBN-13: 978-0-226-71876-7 (cloth)
ISBN-13: 978-0-226-71893-4 (e-book)
DOI: https://doi.org/10.7208/chicago/9780226718934.001.0001

Library of Congress Cataloging-in-Publication Data

Names: Slotten, Ross A., author.
Title: Plague years : a doctor's journey through the AIDS crisis / Ross A. Slotten.
Description: Chicago : University of Chicago Press, 2020.
Identifiers: LCCN 2020004971 | ISBN 9780226718767 (cloth) | ISBN 9780226718934 (ebook)
Subjects: LCSH: AIDS (Disease)—Illinois—Chicago. | AIDS (Disease)
Classification: LCC RA643.84.I3 S568 2020 | DDC 362.19697/9200977311—dc23
LC record available at https://lccn.loc.gov/2020004971

♾ This paper meets the requirements of ANSI/NISO z39.48–1992
(Permanence of Paper).

To those we lost to the AIDS crisis

and to those who survived it

It is a wondrous tale that I have to tell:

if I weren't one of many people who saw it with their own eyes,

I would scarcely have dared to believe it, let alone write it down,

even if I had heard it from a completely trustworthy person ...

— GIOVANNI BOCCACCIO, *The Decameron*

Contents

Prologue

I was there at the beginning of the AIDS epidemic, and I'm still here. I came of age as a doctor and as a gay man during that monumental public health crisis, and thirty-five years later I continue to treat people with or at risk of HIV.

This book is a record of my journey. I kept journals and notes from the first, chronicling the stories of those who died and the few who've survived to the present. Those notes help remind me how and why AIDS ravaged a generation, its impact as catastrophic as that of war and genocide. They also chronicle my own story. My story isn't over yet, and neither is that of AIDS. If we think that it is, we're practically inviting it to run rampant once more.

If my narrative ended in 1995, it would add little to the story of the AIDS epidemic. During the bleakest years, from 1981 until the late 1990s, AIDS sparked a creative outburst in the artistic community, whose members were disproportionately annihilated by the disease and were outraged at the indifference of politicians and policymakers. That output began on the margins but came to include influential mainstream plays, memoirs, films, art installations, two Broadway musicals, and even a symphony. A few straight doctors also reported on their experiences, most notably Abraham Verghese in his classic account *My Own Country*. Once effective treatments became available and the death toll plummeted, a sense of urgency among those afflicted and those who cared for them seemed to dissipate.

But AIDS hasn't disappeared. There is no cure or effective vaccine, so there's no end in sight to one of the worst plagues of modern times. To date, more than seventy-five million people throughout the world have contracted the infection, and thirty-five million have died. Those numbers continue to rise, though no longer at a logarithmic rate. Everyone infected with HIV will carry that virus to their grave, even if what kills them is a heart attack, a stroke, or cancer. But if they stop their lifesaving regimens, known as HAART—highly active antiretroviral therapy—then AIDS will kill them first. Imagine the psychological, physical, and financial burdens a twenty-one-year-old man infected with HIV must shoulder for the next sixty years if no cure is discovered! It takes tremendous discipline and willpower to adhere to a daily therapy you cannot miss. Even though we can now control HIV infection, no one wants it any more than they want to lose their limbs, eyesight, or hearing.

This story marks my progress as a doctor who first confronted a challenge for which nothing could have prepared me and who then unexpectedly became an expert. But more important, it marks stages in our understanding of HIV, beginning before anyone had described AIDS, for the conditions that abetted the spread of the disease were present in the decades before its onset. Epidemics happen for a reason. HIV couldn't have gained a foothold and swept across the world, sparing few places, without the ease of international travel; increased sexual promiscuity brought on by the sexual revolution of the 1960s and 1970s; the rapid spread of other sexually transmitted diseases like gonorrhea, chlamydia, syphilis, herpes, human papilloma virus. and hepatitis A, B, and to a lesser degree C; the failure of political leaders to authorize adequate funding to confront the epidemic in its earliest phases; and the disruption of traditional life in many societies by colonialism and civil wars.

The story I tell here is primarily a Chicago story, for New York, San Francisco, and Los Angeles weren't the only cities whose gay communities were decimated by AIDS. We suffered too, even if the media overlooked us. Because I'm a gay man who treats mainly gay patients, I don't address the epidemic's victims who injected intravenous drugs or were infected through contaminated blood products, or women and children, because those stories are beyond my personal experiences. Those stories are eminently worthy of being told, but the ones I've chosen to tell center on my gay friends and patients. Names and identifying facts have been changed in many instances to protect privacy and maintain confidentiality.

For those who lived through the worst period of the epidemic, this book could bring back memories of an era that we all hope will never be repeated. For those who didn't experience that terrible time, or who've forgotten how terrible it was, let my chapters serve as a warning to the complacent and the ignorant: untreated HIV is as ruthless as any terrorist and as destructive as a nuclear bomb. Humans have *never* conquered any sexually transmitted disease and are unlikely to do so unless they stop having sex. Perhaps HIV will someday become a historical footnote if the infection can be cured or a preventive vaccine is developed, but it won't vanish, just as other sexually transmitted diseases defy eradication despite the earnest efforts of public health officials and medical practitioners. HIV will remain a part of the human landscape for a long time to come.

It's been a privilege for me to travel on this journey with my patients, some of whom have managed to stick with me for more than three decades as the management of their health has evolved and improved dramatically. I hope our collective and separate journeys through a kind of holocaust are worth remembering on their own, and for the lessons they might yet teach.

: 1 :

No End in Sight

(1992)

To the casual visitor, the west wing of the eleventh floor of St. Joseph Hospital didn't look like a vision of hell. The elevator opened into the solarium, a glass-encased semicircular space with a panoramic view of Lincoln Park and Lake Michigan. In the distance sailboats plied the waters beyond a steady stream of traffic on Lake Shore Drive; in the foreground there were joggers on tree-shaded paths. Northward, fashionable high-rises lined the park; to the south rose the iconic skyscrapers of downtown Chicago. What wasn't visible, to the west, was Boys' Town, the city's gayest neighborhood, a jumble of bars, restaurants, sex shops, and inexpensive apartments—the epicenter of the AIDS epidemic in Chicago. It was September 1992, and the city brimmed with life, in stark contrast to 11 West—our AIDS unit—where death reigned.

At 7:00 a.m., when I arrived for hospital rounds, the solarium was usually empty; but occasionally a patient sat staring at the scenic vista, his back to me and his body connected to an intravenous line that snaked from a plastic bag atop a metal pole and disappeared into an arm I could not see; or a patient's lover or family waited for me or one of the other doctors who took care of AIDS patients, seeking an update on their loved one's condition or to ask questions we often couldn't answer. These uncomfortable encounters foreshadowed my visits to the sick and dying patients on the ward. Despite the picturesque urban vista, I could never deceive myself: eleven years into the AIDS epidemic, 11 West was not the place of hope we had conceived of but one of darkness and despair.

Seen from above, St. Joseph Hospital was the shape of an enormous cross, thirteen stories tall. It was a Catholic institution administered by the Daughters of Charity, an order that once commanded the largest nonprofit fleet of hospitals in the United States. The Daughters soft-pedaled their religion. There were, of course, the requisite crucifixes in strategic places, and in the main lobby there was a larger-than-life color photograph of the current pope in full regalia. But everyone was welcome regardless of religious belief (or nonbelief), race, gender, or sexual orientation. During those times when I felt frustrated by our failure to discover life-saving treatments; bristled at the bigotry of evangelists like Jerry Falwell and Pat Robertson, who railed against those infected with HIV as sinners deserving their horrible fate; or struggled with internal demons—guilt about my own good health or rage at my impotence—I sometimes forgot that St. Joe's, as we called it, was a refuge of tolerance and support. But if it hadn't been, it would have been impossible to practice there.

I'd exited the elevators on the eleventh floor so many times during the four years since we'd established 11 West that I rarely bothered to look out the floor-to-ceiling windows. On most days I was in a rush, like most doctors. Pushed and pulled in many directions, I had a lot to accomplish in the two to three hours I could dedicate to rounds. 11 West lay straight ahead, its gleaming linoleum floors forming an elongated truncated triangle. When the doors to the patient rooms were open, they emanated rectangular splashes of light. It reminded me of a runway or stage, but the drama didn't occur in the hallways. It was on the sidelines, in each room, where awful things unfolded.

I stopped at the nurses' station first, gossiping for a few minutes with the unit secretary, Flo or Mary P., and the nurses, like the two Carols, Rita, or Roger, who'd dedicated their professional lives to caring for the patients—mostly gay men of all races and ethnicities from every part of the city and suburbs—who were admitted to, discharged from, readmitted to, or died on the unit. Then I extracted my charts from a carousel and sat down at the long desk, the binders spread out before me like a giant hand of cards. For the next few minutes I caught up on the previous day and night's events, reviewing the notes of the nurses, interns, residents, and consultants, mulling over lab results, and gathering my thoughts about my patients' diagnoses and prognoses.

Doctors are often referred to as healers, or as practitioners of the healing arts. I thought of the two cardiovascular surgeons on staff, who performed lifesaving procedures like cardiac bypass surgery; or my orthopedic friends, who fixed hips and repaired other fractures that in a distant era would have left their patients permanently crippled or deformed. But on 11 West I wasn't healing anyone. I was ministering to my patients, as doctors did in the pre-antibiotic era, doling out bad news, holding a hand in sympathy, or expressing my condolences in the face of an incurable fatal disease. I felt more like a failure than a success, even though HIV-infected gay men from far and wide sought me out because of my expertise and reputation.

As I made my way to the patients' rooms, my shoes clicking on that glistening surface, the pungent odors of sanitizer, shit, and urine—a noxious smell combination unique to hospitals and nursing homes—wafted into my nose. From some of the rooms came sounds of suffering: groans, cries of varying intensities, hacking coughs, vomiting. If I heard laughter, I suspected dementia or an inappropriate response to illness, for there was little to laugh about on 11 West. Rounding on terminally ill patients filled me with intense sadness and wasn't something I looked forward to. My patients hung on to every one of my words and gestures, for what I said or how I said it held the key to their salvation or pointed the way to their demise. It was a pressure almost too much for me to bear.

The first room I entered that morning was that of Troy, a twenty-eight-year-old HIV-infected gay black man, his skin sallow and his head shaved. One week earlier I'd sat on the side of his bed holding his hand as we talked about how he'd get out of the hospital and resume a normal life for a while. I'd been treating him with intravenous antibiotics for a miserable sinus infection, its severity due to his HIV infection, but each day he descended deeper into a depression as he spent more time in bed clutching the left side of his head in pain. On the intended day of discharge, he refused to go home because he still felt terrible, he said, but I couldn't understand why. One week should have been enough time to make inroads against a severe sinus infection, I thought.

Troy had few telltale signs of AIDS—no thrush (a white coating in the mouth and throat caused by a yeast infection); no enlarged lymph nodes; and no purplish lesions of Kaposi's sarcoma, a type of AIDS cancer. His CD4 count, a marker for the state of his immune system, was low but not profoundly low. The absence of such signs had made me too complacent about his health. After examining him and finding nothing wrong, I asked him to stand up. Since his admission, I'd not watched him walk or move about his room; this turned out to have been a serious oversight. Bracing himself on the handrails, he rose from the bed, took a few steps forward, and staggered, which startled me. Laying my hands on his shoulders, I kept him from falling to the ground as it dawned on me that he was suffering from something more serious than sinusitis and depression. And he was. The next day he had a seizure and lost consciousness. A CAT scan of his brain showed multiple tumors, diffuse disease of the white matter, and swelling of the brain, images suggesting that his death was imminent. I'd not suspected the grave diagnosis—brain lymphoma—so convinced was I that something more benign was causing his headaches and fatigue (an x-ray of his sinuses had indeed shown sinusitis). Miraculously, he improved after I prescribed high doses of steroids, which alleviated pressure on the part of the brainstem that controlled his vital functions. But that was temporary.

Several days after the seizure I found Troy alert but debilitated by severe neurological deficits. His room was dark except for a television blasting inanities. In the flickering artificial light he lay on his back with his neck twisted awkwardly to the left ("looking at the brain lesions," as the consulting neurologist, Dr. L., explained) like someone who'd had a stroke. His lower lip protruded, and he breathed through his mouth, but both lips were scaly and cracked. His face glistened with oily secretions from the pores, and he smelled of urine and sweat despite the nurses' best efforts to keep him clean. How much had changed in so short a time, I thought. A vibrant young man seemed to have aged fifty years in the space of two weeks. Pity gripped me as I approached the bedside, but as a doctor I had learned to suppress emotions, for they can cloud clinical judgment and lead to faulty decisions. A sick person wants to see strength in his doctor, not weakness, although too much suppression makes the doctor seem cold and uncaring. Each time I confronted a dying patient, or any patient for that matter, I struggled to find the right balance between compassion and aloofness; this struggle took place scores of times every day. The internal conflict manifests itself in my journals, where "one" and "you" often replaces the more personal "I." Unconsciously I gave myself permission to detach from my true feelings and excuse myself from taking responsibility for painful decisions and actions. I know this now, after decades of reflection.

Pulling up a chair, I sat down beside the head of the bed, took Troy's hand, and called his name.

"Hello," Troy responded in a garbled voice, unable to turn his head toward me.

The muscles on the right side of his neck seemed to bulge because of the strain on the left. With his neck bent in such a vulnerable way, he reminded me of a sacrificial lamb waiting to be slaughtered. An impairment of his eye muscles made each eye rove separately and prevented him from looking at me directly. Although when I asked him to he squeezed my fingers with his left hand, indicating higher cognitive function, he couldn't move the rest of his arm. I asked myself if this was the best he'd ever be and concluded it probably was. What a nightmare! I should never have tried to treat him, I lamented inside. It would have been best to let him die rather than keep him in the hospital to languish in such a dependent state for the remaining days or weeks of his life. I didn't tell him this because it was my job to give some degree of hope even in the most hopeless situations. Yet given the severity of his disability, it wasn't possible to have a meaningful conversation with him. All I could do was pat him on the shoulder, grope for a few reassuring if meaningless words, and move on. And so I did.

The next patient I visited was a man named Robert, who suffered from an AIDS-related brain infection known as PML (progressive multifocal leukoencephalopathy). Like Troy's, his head was twisted to the left, which was only a coincidence, for the young men suffered from different brain diseases. Each time I stopped in his room during rounds, he recognized me, even when I thought he couldn't see me; it was as if he had a sixth sense. At the sight or sound of me, or anyone, he reared up stiff as a rocking horse, head arcing forward, knees bowed toward his face. Despite the devastating brain infection, he had complete control over his mental faculties. Before his illness, Robert had performed in the chorus of a major opera company. Now dozens of get-well cards from fellow artists and friends cluttered the room; cards had been taped to the curtains that divided his space from that of another AIDS patient. Vases of flowers had transformed the dreary windowsill into a miniature greenhouse. A note on the dresser beside his bed begged the staff not to remove a ribbon pinned to his gown (it was a symbol from his church), but I'd not seen it in days. A copy of *Opera News* lay unopened on a chair.

A once corpulent black man, Robert had withered nearly into a skeleton. When I first met him, he had been something of a bon vivant. He loved to tell stories, and it was a pleasure listening to his rich baritone voice—he all but trilled at the ends of sentences. He told me once about a rehearsal of an opera, *Der Rosenkavalier*, by the German composer Richard Strauss. As he sang, he had flung out his arms, inadvertently striking one of the leading sopranos, who had a notorious reputation for confrontation and ill-temper, in the face. The conductor stopped the orchestra, and several painful seconds passed as everyone on stage froze in horror. Mortified and expecting to be fired on the spot, Robert apologized profusely; but, unhurt, the soprano waved him off with a smile, and the rehearsal continued. *Trill!*

Now, although he didn't have a fever, Robert's brow was beaded with sweat. As he drooled, an unpleasant odor wafted from his mouth, like the acrid smell of old blood. Unable to control the movements of his arms and legs, he couldn't hold a cup or plastic urinal. A Foley catheter had been inserted into his penis to prevent him from soiling himself. The skin of his thighs, calves, and feet, taut with fluid, looked like shiny shellacked table legs. He asked me for a glass of water. In fact, he ritualistically asked every visitor for water. Refusing a straw, he drank at a glacial pace. I could hear him swallow in loud gulps, but the water level in the glass barely changed. Water fell onto his chest in droplets, which I mopped up with a washcloth. After drinking, he mumbled "Thank you," then asked me, in a tremulous tone that was a mere echo of the magisterial voice of his more robust days, when he'd be able to walk again like the AIDS patients he observed walking up and down the halls.

"Robert, you won't walk," I said. "If it were pneumocystis or CMV we could treat it and you'd get better, but there is no treatment for your problem. I'm afraid this is the best things will be. I know it's horrible."

The words sounded cruel to me, but I couldn't lie to him, for nothing would reverse the progress of his disease. Robert paused for the longest time, pondering my statement. When gauging someone's thoughts, we depend on facial expressions and body language for clues to inner feelings, but Robert's PML had destroyed those physical cues. I guessed that he was bewildered or shocked, as if I'd told him about his illness for the first time. After an excruciating silence, he asked me when he could go home. I had to tell him that he couldn't go home without around-the-clock care, which was beyond his means. Although he had a large group of friends, no one could make that kind of commitment, I said. And his mother, a sweet but frail woman in Louisville, Kentucky, was overwhelmed by her son's medical condition. After spending a week in Chicago at his bedside, she had returned home for a few days but planned to take a leave of absence from work to help care for him. But even with the assistance of home hospice, I couldn't imagine her lifting him or carrying him to the bathroom or helping him into a wheelchair every day for weeks or months. Like Troy, he would most likely remain in the hospital until his death.

The third patient I rounded on was Steve, who'd suffered during the last few months from intractable diarrhea, advancing Kaposi's sarcoma, CMV retinitis, and neuropathy—one devastating AIDS-related problem after another. His lover Sean confided to me that at home he exploded in fits of rage, which upset Sean and their roommate Heather. On a previous admission he'd groaned all night, his nurse Rita had reported, but he told me that he was "all right." I knew he wasn't. Should he give up or go on? he asked at every visit. He wanted to do both but couldn't decide. Before becoming ill, he had worked as an artistic director at an advertising firm. He had been a handsome, tall, lanky white man. Now a beaklike nose jutted out from a gaunt face. His eyes sank into their sockets, and when he slept they remained half open like those of a corpse. Patches of hair were all that remained of his once luxuriant mane. When healthy, he had been self-conscious about his psoriasis, which spared his face but erupted in red scaly plaques on his torso, extremities, and penis. As he became more immune suppressed, his psoriasis had all but disappeared, for reasons I couldn't explain. What replaced the psoriasis was far worse. He had the papery tan skin of a mummy. In fact, his whole lower body was mummified. Kaposi's sarcoma had turned his legs into purple-brown carapaces and bloated his feet like those of a dead body floating in a river.

Sean had brought him to the hospital initially because of a severe headache, but after a thorough workup I couldn't identify a specific cause, and never would. One day he became confused and began mumbling. Restless, he grasped and picked at the sheets like someone with a severe obsessive-compulsive disorder. When I'd spoken to Sean earlier in the week, before Steve's final hospitalization, he said he wanted it "straight" and used a tough-guy tone inflected with a Boston accent—many of us gay men in those days went to great lengths to appear more masculine, or butch, in the eyes of a disapproving world. When I gave it to him straight, he cried. He knew that Steve's condition was hopeless, but he couldn't let Steve go. That morning he stood at the bedside gripping the guardrails and sagging in despair. He followed me out of the room to ask more questions, beyond Steve's earshot. Hugging him as he sobbed into my coat, I fought off my own tears, unable to imagine how I would react if my own boyfriend verged on death. In normal circumstances we'd be elderly, our sorrow no less painful but mitigated by the knowledge that we'd lived long lives and our time had come. We were all too young to be dealing with such monumental issues.

I marvel how people can hold on to the thinnest thread of hope when the only outcome, death, is obvious, I reflected in my journal that night. My partner of nine years, Gavin, had already fallen asleep in the bedroom of our townhouse, but sleep eluded me. I sat in bed by the lamplight and scribbled down whatever thoughts came to mind without attempting to interpret what I'd experienced that day.

It's as if a person is clinging to a cliff. You clutch both hands but one hand slips away. As you tighten the grip on the other, it too slips away. In desperation you grab a piece of clothing, but that piece rips off. The person falls screaming and all you're left with is a fragment of cloth. And still you believe the person is somehow alive. All three of the patients are cloth fragments, I think. You can't classify them as living. They breathe; they sweat; they urinate; they shit—the only evidence of life. Otherwise, they're in the land of the dead. They reek of death—from the skin, from the breath, from the rectum, from the interstices of their human shell. The stink of AIDS, which stinks like no other disease I know. Each death from a particular disease has its own stink. AIDS patients rot from the inside out, though they often rot from the outside in. When they breathe, the rot pours out, like the smell of waste from a sewer. Their bodies are sewers. Death for them is rarely peaceful or beautiful. It's a relief!

But whose relief was I referring to? The patients', the families' and friends', or my own? I felt so weary, in some ways as helpless as all three of these men. I was a caregiver who shepherded his patients from the land of the living to the land of the dead, like the boatman Charon, ferryman to Hades—not the role I'd envisioned as an enthusiastic, idealistic twenty-seven-year-old man with the newly minted initials MD after my name when I graduated from medical school in June 1981. As an intern, unlike as a medical student, I was in charge of my patients, which I had found exhilarating. In consultation with each patient's private physician and my supervising senior resident, I had learned how to manage all sorts of patient problems, modeling my bedside manner on that of doctors I admired, while noting and striving to avoid the bad traits in those I didn't. Most of those patients went home, better off than when they were admitted, inflating my ego and my sense of self-worth. Now more than a decade had passed since the first cases of AIDS had been identified in the United States. In June 1981, a few weeks before I began my internship in family practice at St. Joe's, the Center for Disease Control in Atlanta had published the first report of a strange lethal infection among a cohort of gay men in Los Angeles. I had no clue then that the disease would soon kill friends, former lovers, colleagues, and patients; devastate tens of millions of people and their families worldwide; and consume my entire professional life and more than half my chronological one.

In 1984 I opened a practice with Tom K., who'd completed his training in family medicine at St. Joe's three years before I did. Our office was in a nondescript building called Seton Medical Center on the north side of Chicago, on the margins of two historic neighborhoods: Old Town, once the haunt of artists, writers, intellectuals, and other eccentrics; and Cabrini Green, one of the most notorious housing projects in the nation, overrun by gangs but also home to hardworking people who had trouble finding affordable housing because of their race and low income. The Daughters of Charity had bought a vacant garbage-filled lot spanning more than half a block from the city for a low price because it was their laudable mission to build medical clinics in underserved areas.

Seton's location was a boon to Tom and me because we both had obligations to the National Health Service Corps, which had funded our medical education. That scholarship, established in the early 1970s, encouraged newly trained doctors to pursue a career in primary care instead of one of the more lucrative specialties like oph-thalmology, radiology, or anesthesia. Healthcare planners feared a shortage of family physicians and internists. The scholarship spared us from the mountain of debt many young doctors faced. And I earned some extra money from side jobs (drawing blood from patients admitted to Lakeside VA at Northwestern, where I had at-tended medical school; performing histories and physicals on patients scheduled for routine surgery; moonlighting in the emer-gency department at St. Joe's), and this allowed me to indulge one of my passions, international travel. That provoked my father to jest that I spent four years in medical school and one year touring the world.

Ordinarily the National Health Service Corps would have as-signed Tom and me to positions in the Indian Health Service or rural America, which were in desperate need of primary care doc-tors because they were remote and poverty-stricken. Only some sort of draft would bring doctors to them, for few of us volunteered to go there. But Ronald Reagan, whom we otherwise despised for his public homophobia and failure to address the AIDS crisis be-fore it spiraled out of control, created the so-called private practice option that allowed young doctors like us more freedom of choice. As long as we practiced in an underserved area and agreed to see patients who were uninsured or on Medicaid, we could remain in Chicago. At first our practice attracted people from the two neigh-borhoods, but we went one step further: our office soon became a refuge for people marginalized for reasons other than race, mainly men who had nowhere else to go or who had been kicked out of the previous doctors' practices because they were gay, had AIDS, or were at risk of AIDS.

By 1984 Tom had made a name for himself in the Chicago gay community through his volunteer work at Howard Brown Memo-rial Clinic, which treated gay men near the heart of Boys' Town. With his encouragement, I'd been volunteering there too. Tom was a big man with a big personality, his cherubic face framed by perfectly coiffed chestnut hair and a neatly trimmed beard. His patients adored him, and he had a wide circle of friends. With his charm and ease in a variety of social settings, in another life he could have been a successful politician. Raised in a conservative Dutch Reformed household in suburban Detroit, he was far less reticent about being gay than I, whose parents were liberal secular Jews in suburban Chicago. Although his mother and father had come to terms with his sexual orientation after years of confusion and anguish, others in his extended family continued to sneer at what they viewed as a sinful life; a great-aunt had sent him a greeting card consigning him to hell. For me the journey to full acceptance would take many years, long after I became a respected AIDS specialist.

In the beginning Tom and I weren't the only AIDS doctors in town. There were a handful of others, like the two Davids at Illinois Masonic Hospital, Bernie B. at Rush, Tom C. at Northwestern, Michael B. at Weiss Hospital, and a few others who didn't survive the early days of the epidemic. As gay men, we felt that it was our duty to serve the gay community, which bore the brunt—and continues to bear the brunt—of the AIDS crisis, not only in Chicago but elsewhere in the United States, for two-thirds of people with HIV in this part of the world were and are gay men. Although Chicago is a segregated city—a white North Side and black South Side—AIDS in the 1980s was not a North Side–South Side issue. In the close-knit gay community, patients of all ethnicities and races from every neighborhood found sympathetic, dedicated gay doctors to care for them. Although we also treated small numbers of heterosexual patients who'd acquired HIV through intravenous drug use or blood transfusions, as well as women who'd contracted HIV from a bisexual partner, their numbers paled in comparison to the number of HIV-infected gay men. We didn't turn away those who weren't gay, but most HIV-infected heterosexual men and women knew nothing about our office and wound up elsewhere, like Cook County Hospital, where our good friends Ron S. and Renslow S. had set up a clinic and the city's first AIDS unit.

Tom and I might never have become AIDS specialists had St. Joe's employed a full-time infectious disease expert in the critical years between 1984 and 1986. The absence of such a specialist forced us to learn how to diagnose and treat the ailing men who streamed into our practice as best we could. By 1986 St. Joe's had hired Roberta L., an infectious disease specialist who became a dear friend and fellow combatant in this hideous war, but by that time we'd embraced our role as pioneers in a new field of medicine and no longer needed to refer patients to a specialist. In 1992, as I wrote those entries in my journal, I had the dubious distinction of having signed more death certificates in the city of Chicago—and by inference the entire state of Illinois—than any other physician. How many deaths had I witnessed; how many more could I withstand before breaking down?

I had no answers to such questions. In fact, such questions eluded my mind that morning in September as I finished my rounds, recorded my observations and recommendations in my patients' charts, and returned to the elevators without acknowledging the beautiful urban landscape outside the windows. Lost in thought, I descended to the first floor, stored my gray coat in a locker in the doctors' lounge, chatted with colleagues, exited the hospital for the garage, slipped into my car, and headed to my office. But once in the car, with a few moments alone, the enormity of what I'd confronted tormented me.

How close we always are, I think, to death, I wrote that day, recording what I felt as I drove through neighborhoods where people went about their business seemingly untouched by the AIDS epidemic. They hadn't the slightest inkling of what my patients and I were experiencing—they lived in a different world from mine, oblivious to the humanitarian catastrophe at their doorsteps. *I live life as if the precipice is continually on one side of me. One step and I'm over and done with. Often I have that same sensation you have when you are on top of a mountain, looking over the edge. An invisible force presses against you, to keep you from falling. A momentary vertigo as you fathom the abyss. That thrill of being so close to death. Yes, a thrill, which is the obverse of fear. Your breath stops mid-way. What keeps me from throwing myself off? I wonder. All these feelings are encapsulated in the moment when I ponder death and I think of my patients dying. That force against my chest, that abrupt halting of the breath.*

Sometimes I wondered what kept me from throwing myself off the precipice, either literally or figuratively. Perhaps it was my idealistic sense of duty and refusal to abandon my community during its darkest hour; or the adrenaline rush I experienced from being at the forefront of a new field of medicine, which exaggerated my importance in my own eyes and the eyes of my patients and colleagues; or the instinctive drive for self-preservation, which prevented me from having a nervous breakdown or, worse, committing suicide; or simply inertia, because maintaining the status quo, terrible as it was, seemed less frightening to me than change, such as pursuing a different career in medicine. Questioning motives sows doubt; doubt leads to indecision; and indecision to inaction, the worst possible response to a crisis, especially for a doctor. So I simply did not question my motives.

Others might have turned to a pastor or rabbi to address such quandaries, but religion was a foreign language I never learned. Synagogues, mosques, and churches didn't (and still don't) inspire feelings of reverence in me, although I respect those for whom they do. When seated in a pew or temple chair, I feel like a trespasser or tourist. Although my parents identified as Jews, they didn't practice any sort of religion; they described themselves as agnostics. My mother skipped Hebrew school classes and intercepted letters to her parents reporting her truancy until an older sister ratted on her. After his bar mitzvah, my father stopped going to synagogue. My mother eventually explained to me that she didn't feel comfortable compelling us to do something she didn't do or, as in my father's case, did reluctantly. As a result I grew up an atheist whose moral compass was defined not by religious dogma but my parents' moral code, which essentially adhered to the Golden Rule but without an angry God to reinforce it.

Each day of my life during those dark times, I searched for some way to move forward. Days spilled into weeks, weeks into months, and months into years as the AIDS epidemic ground on. I wasn't the only one grappling with these issues. There were tens of thousands of us throughout the country and world: public health officials; scientific and clinical researchers; doctors, nurses, physician assistants; and other caregivers, all of us dedicated to a single cause. We intersected at international, national, and local conferences, creating a network that laid the groundwork for finding some solution to the AIDS crisis, of whatever form. When that crisis would end, and how we would survive emotionally and professionally in the intervening time of uncertainty, none of us could fathom.

: 2 :

First Cairn

(1984)

For all my interest in gay men's health, most of the patients I saw in my office in the first year of practice, 1984, were heterosexual. I filled my journals with descriptions of elderly men and women who came to me through the emergency department, often when I was moonlighting there (in those days you didn't have to be board certified in Emergency Medicine to work in an ED). An ambulance had whisked them to St. Joe's even if their primary care physicians were on staff at different hospitals. By law, the fire department had to bring patients to the hospital nearest their home. I admit that even from my earliest days in practice I had a weakness for old people. I did everything in my power to woo them, including making home visits after their discharge. Perhaps they reminded me of the grandparents I never took the time to get to know during my adolescence, when I was too self-absorbed to care about anyone but me.

I kept journals because I fantasized that one day I would be a famous writer. In the early days I had no subject. It was important to write, write, and write, like a painter learning to paint. In college I had taken a creative writing course and dabbled in fiction. I read many of the great fiction writers—Tolstoy, Dostoyevsky, Mann, and Proust (all seven volumes) were among my early favorites. In those days I was such a fucking snob! Perhaps I still am. But I soon realized that I lacked the imagination to write a novel or short story. Soon I gravitated toward nonfiction. I read Darwin's *Origin of Species* between my freshman and sophomore years and became a committed evolutionist. Decades later I would publish a biography of the man who formulated the theory of natural selection independently of Darwin, Alfred Russel Wallace; but in the 1970s that was an unforeseen outcome.

One journal covers my first journey to Europe in 1977 after graduating from college, with sketches included, just like those of nineteenth-century travelers making a similar rite of passage. In my childhood we had never traveled internationally; in fact we rarely ventured beyond the Midwest. Extended travel was impossible because my father took only five days off a year. Once when I was ten years old—several months after John F Kennedy was assassinated—we drove to Washington, DC: two days there—four kids loaded into a bench seat in the back of the station wagon, my parents up front; one day to see the sites; one long day back. It was on this trip that I somehow learned to whistle—and I'm now a very good whistler with a strong vibrato—at my father's encouragement and patient instruction. My mother kept a journal, which we all happily contributed to, but it's lost. Perhaps inspired by that effort, I continued to journal on my own but with no clear plan for what I would do with its contents.

I met Mrs. Cook *on the very last paragraph of her long life (90 years!)*, as I put it in my journal from 1984. At first she looked like every other old lady I saw in the hospital or on the streets. Her face had less range of emotional expression because of diminished mobility (a flat affect, as psychiatrists called it), and her unique personality wasn't apparent. But after talking to her, I realized that she harbored strong convictions. When emphasizing a point, she squeezed my hands, looking me right in the eye with an expression of defiance mixed with a yearning for love and affection. Having lived so many years, she said, she wanted to share her most instructive experiences with those of us who were young and striking out into the world. She made it clear that I was to be not simply her doctor but also a friend. Given a week, she would have recounted everything; but during rounds I had only a few minutes to lend an ear.

Mrs. Cook boasted about all the young people who flocked to her and sought her wisdom. Her hairdresser Ron, for example, came to her apartment to cut her hair and confided "very personal things" to her. She accepted his homosexuality and adored him like a grandson. Here was an opportunity for my own confession, but I prevaricated and nodded with admiration at her open-mindedness. Professionally I still lived a closeted life.

Between long hours of clarity Mrs. Cook had her mental lapses. She would argue endlessly with her son and daughter about her drinking problem. It seemed that a carafe of brandy would be emptied in one or two days. She insisted that she only took "nips" now and then to help her breathe and settle her stomach. They also chided her about her smoking, but she denied smoking more than one or two cigarettes a day. In my presence she polished off five or six. When reaching a climax in a conversation, she would grunt and groan as if gasping for breath or preparing to vomit. Then she would get restless and pace, unable to articulate what she was feeling. Her abdomen became distended and she belched a lot; but if she had her daily bowel movement, without which she would never be quite right, she said, her symptoms improved. On my first encounter of the alarming scene of her distension, I feared her death was imminent. But after a burp or a fart she recovered.

Despite her age, she was still a sexual being and would make remarks that startled me, like referring to her cunt or hoping to get laid. In those early days of my career, I failed to realize how important sex is to the elderly; it was as if I thought the idea of sex disappears at some particular day or time, like menopause or qualifying for Medicare. When an octogenarian broached the topic, somehow I thought he or she was being "cute" and I laughed — just as I might laugh when a three-year-old says something precocious — having never considered that the desire for sex, like the lust for life, doesn't end until your final breath.

Not long before she died, I visited her apartment at the request of her daughter. She'd developed a small-cell cancer of the lung, and both lungs were riddled with tumors. Because small-cell cancers respond to chemotherapy, she agreed to treatment. Afterward the tumors seemed to have vanished. But "something wasn't quite right," her daughter said. Her mother refused to leave her apartment; she hadn't ventured out in months except for treatment. Now she wouldn't even do that. Fatiguing easily, she complained of abdominal pain and "pissing all over herself," the unpredictability of which was one of the main reasons for staying home.

Although the building she lived in was a bright new brick highrise on the fringe of the Gold Coast, her apartment, decorated in fleecy grays and dull browns, belonged to an older era. The furniture had had an antique flavor even when purchased in the 1920s or 1930s. The glassware resembled prisms—it wasn't sleek Finnish ware but the type seen in daguerreotypes or old European films. Dust puffed out of the carpets, and a haze of cigarette smoke choked the air. The ammonia odor of urine mixed with smoke and dust burned my nostrils. My father's parents had a similar taste in interior design, but they were also obsessively neat, which Mrs. Cook was not. It surprised me that her children tolerated this degree of squalor, but Mrs. Cook was headstrong and allowed no one, especially her children, to interfere with her life.

I held her hand as she spoke, looking at the parchmentlike skin and cords of veins that disappeared up the sleeve of her blouse. In comparison, my hands were pink and plump, the veins hidden within youthful flesh. She no longer bothered to color her hair, which was short and unkempt; mine, which was neat, lacked even a fleck of grey. Gnarled toes protruded from her slippers and dried urine stained her nightgown. At that moment, gazing at her weary face, I felt more like her grandson than her doctor—like a child in a lab coat. I couldn't find much wrong when I listened to her lungs and heart. Her pulse was strong and regular, and blood pressure was normal—or at least I couldn't detect any new worrisome signs of a dangerous illness or recurrence of her cancer. Before I left she asked for a hug, and I promised to visit her again soon.

A few days after my visit Mrs. Cook died at home, suddenly but peacefully. Although her death wasn't unexpected, I was caught off guard. Although she had lived to be ninety and had cancer, I still felt that somehow I'd failed her. Her daughter had sensed that something was wrong, but I'd missed whatever it was. Was that failure due to inexperience, I wondered, or incompetence? I found it hard not to feel despondent, not only about her death but also about my inadequacy as a physician. But I wasn't a failure or inept. Just three years in as a licensed physician, I was inexperienced. And I was not inured to life's harshest reality: death.

My first intimate experience of human death had occurred in anatomy class in 1977. As a child and adolescent I'd known something of death: an aunt had died of breast cancer; a kid in my brother's grammar-school class had been killed in a bicycle accident; a neighbor had lost a battle with lung cancer; and a friend of a friend had been stabbed to death on my college campus one summer. But up to the time of this class, the death of a beloved person remained a theoretical concept. I'd never grieved the death of any human being, only that of a guinea pig named Peter whom I spoiled from the ages of six to twelve and buried in a shoebox in our backyard, with a stake to mark the spot and a promise never to forget my cherished childhood companion.

In anatomy class, as we rolled out the cadaver from its refrigerated crypt and unwrapped the plastic encasement, I got goosebumps. Here was a dead person, naked and old. The pungent odor of formaldehyde distracted me from my discomfort. There were four of us in my dissection group, two standing on each side of the body. We said nothing as we contemplated the elderly black woman whose personal history we didn't know. Had she been married? Had she worked? We would soon learn whether she'd had children. I marveled that this woman had donated her body to science. I asked myself if I would do the same, but I had no answer. It was impossible to think that far into the future or consider my own death.

The dean, an ex-hippie not much older than I who kayaked every day from his home in Evanston to downtown Chicago—more than ten miles—lectured us about treating our cadavers with respect, as if he were a priest chastising a flock of sinners. Under pain of immediate suspension or expulsion, he said, we were not to play pranks like jumping rope with the intestines or tossing body parts at each other. A few people stifled laughs. Until he mentioned it, it would never have occurred to me to jump rope with an intestine. Why was he telling us this? Because it *had* occurred to someone there once. In retrospect, I recognized that this was our first lesson in medical ethics, which is nothing more than the Golden Rule, the one I grew up with: Do unto others as you would have them do unto you.

On the first day of dissection, some people fainted. I didn't; I felt awe-inspired. Death wasn't the subject of anatomy; life was. We analyzed every aspect of our cadaver so that we could understand how each organ system functioned, in health and in disease. I memorized the names of arteries, veins, and nerves; isolated each muscle; and examined the skeleton. In short, I learned what made humans human. At first it amused me when the chief of pathology, a forensic pathologist, lectured to us about his "patients." A short and unintentionally funny man with bushy, mobile eyebrows and exaggerated hand movements, he could never convince me that his so-called patients were anything more than anonymous corpses on whom he performed autopsies. I didn't appreciate that these individuals, who had lived and loved as much as anyone until their lives ended, meant as much to him as the people I cared for would later mean to me.

I witnessed my first death in medical school during a cardiac arrest, as doctors, nurses, and technicians swarmed around a patient—unknown to most of them—to try to resuscitate him. At the time I could do nothing but observe a process that was both orderly in its adherence to protocol and chaotic because of the number of people involved. We'd shock the heart with electrified paddles, causing the body to jump like a ragdoll, push oxygen into lungs through a tube, pump the patient with a variety of chemicals to keep the heart going if we conjured a heartbeat, prop up the blood pressure, and pour in fluids through one or more veins to keep the kidneys from shutting down. Sometimes we "worked on" the person, as we put it, for a long time until the attending physician ordered a stop to the heroics. Other times, when a case seemed hopeless yet an attending physician urged us onward, interns and residents mumbled their frustration, but no one dared to object. The focus was on staving off death for as long as possible.

Throughout my training, I responded to numerous cardiac arrests, or "code blues." When "code blue, code blue, room such-and-such" blared from the loudspeakers, I dropped what I was doing and rushed to assist. When it was over, I'd return to the task the code had interrupted and move on, as if nothing momentous had happened. I might even have eaten a sandwich—as an intern and resident, I often ate on the fly.

I had few role models to teach me how to talk with a dying person, how to present treatment options, how to know when to stop treatment, and how to help the patient let go of life. In general, my instructors did a poor job of confronting death and dying; we had no lectures about end-of-life issues. If a patient died, you had somehow failed. When a doctor had to tell someone that no further treatment would extend or improve the quality of life, he or she was often cold or brusque. That brusqueness often wasn't hardheartedness but masked deep feelings of failure that they were repressing. Still, at the worst moment in their lives, patients rarely got any display of warmth, like holding a hand, giving a hug, shedding a tear, or telephoning a few days later to demonstrate concern. Our instructors frowned upon touching a patient in this way, deeming it unprofessional.

When I was an intern, one of the attending family physicians introduced the concept of "orthonasia," a term he'd invented for the management of a dying patient. In euthanasia you take an active role in ending a person's life, an idea that violates the original Hippocratic Oath ("Nor shall any man's entreaty prevail upon me to administer poison to anyone"), though the abridged "modern-day" oath I took during my graduation ceremony does not address it directly ("The health of my patient will be my first consideration"). According to my mentor, orthonasia meant you did nothing but let nature take its course. The concept seemed logical to me—but someone had to present that idea to the patient or the patient's family. Since in this case the patient wasn't my mentor's patient, the discussion, while thought-provoking, remained hypothetical.

During my residency, one death haunted me. It occurred on a rotation in the intensive care unit. The patient, a middle-aged man who had some form of leukemia, had failed to respond to therapy. One of the chemotherapy drugs blistered his gastrointestinal tract, from mouth to anus. Blood oozed from every orifice. Unable to breathe because of the disease, he'd been placed on a ventilator. Conscious despite large doses of sedatives, he begged to stop all treatments. But his doctor, an oncologist, wouldn't let go. In a state of denial, she believed that his life could be saved; nothing would dissuade her. His death struck me as among the most miserable and agonizing I'd ever seen. I vowed never to be the type of doctor who refuses to respect the wishes of a dying patient.

At this time in my career, the hospital patients I cared for who died weren't my patients or my responsibility. The attending physician decided the course of care; I implemented the orders. Mrs. Cook was different. She was my patient and my responsibility. I'd spent months getting to know her and had developed a relationship with her. As she wished, I'd become her friend as well as her doctor. As her friend, I avoided the topic of death so as not to upset her; as her doctor, I neglected to engage her in a meaningful discussion of her mortality. I didn't ask whether she wanted to be resuscitated if her heart stopped or whether we should eschew artificial life support and ease her into death with a pain reliever like morphine. I kept putting off the discussion for another day, the time never seemed right, and she avoided the subject too, except in passing, as if it were a joke. Just as when she mentioned sex, I squirmed with discomfort at the thought of having a heart-to-heart talk about her death. In this regard I was no better than the oncologist I disapproved of. It wasn't that I failed to respect Mrs. Cook's wishes; I just didn't bother to find out what they were.

Her daughter called me to give me the news. I expressed my condolences and told her how much I liked her mother. I was sorry

I couldn't have done more for her, I said. She replied that her mother's death was a relief and a blessing, and she thanked me for my attentive care and making her mother's final days a bit brighter.

For me, Mrs. Cook's death marked the first cairn in a long line of cairns up a professional mountain. She was the first patient I lost after starting my private practice. Because she died at home in her sleep, I'd managed to skirt the big issues. The next time, and other times after, it might not be so easy. I knew even at that early point in my career that if I was going to become a more effective physician, I had to do more than diagnose and treat illnesses. I had to learn how to confront death.

: 3 :

Out of the Closet
and into the Fire
(Before 1983)

I n early March 1985, less than a year after I had completed my training as a family physician, my ex-lover Art called our office because he had diarrhea. Although Art was Tom's patient—I'd referred him—pink slips with messages from all of our patients were posted on a board in the lab area that both of us could see. When I read this one, I didn't think twice about the complaint. As long as I'd known him, Art had had an obsession with his bowels. It wasn't unusual for him to have five or six loose stools a day. But in April he began to ask for Lomotil, a potent antidiarrheal agent that contains a small dose of an opiate, a distant relative of heroin. Soon he was calling several times a week to refill his prescription.

When he came to the office for a checkup in May, two years had passed since I'd last seen him. His face looked gaunt and his clothes hung loosely on his frame, but except for the diarrhea, he said that he felt well. He still sported a thick, trimmed mustache, but his hair had thinned into a tonsure. Oversized glasses framed the blue eyes that had attracted me to him originally. I gave him an obligatory hug and exchanged brief pleasantries, as if nothing more intimate had ever passed between us. In that fleeting moment, all memories, good and bad, vanished. After he entered the exam room and the door closed behind him, some of those memories and others from my past flooded back.

I'd met Art in the fall of 1978 at Alfie's, one of the hottest gay bars in Chicago, on Rush Street a few blocks west of the Northwestern medical school campus. Although fashionable today in the 2000s, in the late 1970s and early 1980s Rush Street had some of the raunchiest bars and clubs in the city. It attracted tourists and the hoi polloi. During the day the building looked abandoned; it came to life at night. Sometimes I'd circle Alfie's a few times until I worked up the nerve to go in. Feeling full of shame, I looked in every direction to make sure no one from the medical center was there to recognize me. It was a ridiculous precaution: only another gay man — or someone wishing to harm a gay man — would venture to Alfie's.

Because of persistent prejudice and hostility, many gay bars had no windows, and doormen guarded the entrances to keep out gay-bashers. The thick door at Alfie's barely muffled the thumping disco music, and the scent of cigarette smoke seeped out. Inside it was dark, smoky, and deafening. Most men went to bars to hook up with someone, but I wasn't looking for anonymous sex. I went hoping to find a long-term partner. I hated cruising, which meant standing in a corner or against a wall making eye contact with the hundreds of men who streamed by. The ear-shattering music killed casual conversation; you had to shout into someone's ear to be understood, and that kind of verbal exchange didn't last long. To distract myself and disguise my nervousness, I would sip a beer without gusto. Often I went home alone and disappointed.

It had taken me a few painful years to get even to this point. Back when I had grappled with the academic requirements to get into medical school, I was also grappling with my sexual identity. I wasted a good deal of my college years at Stanford University, from 1972 to 1976, in varying states of confusion about who or what I was. Several friends have told me that they knew they were gay, even as young children. In high school I had no doubt that I was attracted to women. I had a girlfriend. We made out. Years later I learned that she was a lesbian. That conviction about being heterosexual (the terms *straight* and *gay* hadn't entered my vocabulary) persisted in college until my senior year.

My roommate that year was a tall, handsome African American man named Neal, who was flamboyant, extroverted, and self-confident, my opposite on the personality scale. We met on day one in our dorm's lounge when we were asked to select roommates during an introductory meeting. He zeroed in on me, perhaps because of gaydar—that innate sense gay men have about others who might be gay but don't yet know it—and I didn't resist because he was charismatic. At first I worried that his wardrobe, like his personality, would overwhelm mine. But we turned out to be a perfect match, like Felix and Oscar from the odd couple, and equally humorous. When listening to a song by Chaka Khan or some other black pop singer who meant nothing to me (my musical tastes were strictly classical at the time), he'd amuse me by wagging a finger to make a point or lip-synching lyrics. We'd talk long into the night about everything, from coursework to what it was like to be a black student on a mainly white campus to the antics of our housemates. The one subject we skirted was sexuality. Neal hinted at his proclivities but, uncertain of mine, remained evasive about his sex life. But he loved to, as he said, "par-tay." He'd go out on the weekends somewhere and return high or drunk. I suspect that he spent a lot of time in San Francisco, and he would have regaled me with stories had I asked. I didn't ask. And I didn't "par-tay." On a Saturday night you'd find me in a library, studying.

Years later, Neal told me that he was the first to point out to my girlfriend, Chris, that I might be gay since we never progressed beyond the half-dressed phase, much to her frustration. He also revealed to me the breadth of gay life on campus while we'd been at Stanford. On his telling almost everyone was gay, which was an exaggeration, but he startled me when he listed the names of gay students, administrators, and faculty members with whom I had frequently associated. It was a Proustian underworld in which all the characters you thought you knew revealed themselves to be something entirely different. Decades later, I now wonder how many of these men survived the coming conflagration.

Since I completed my premedical requirements only during my senior year (I'd wandered academically, obtaining a degree in classics before one in biology), I had to delay entry into medical school until the fall of 1977. For nine months I worked in a lab at the Stanford Medical Center for a pediatrician who researched the effects of a virus called CMV (cytomegalovirus) on newborn babies. During that time I shared a house in Palo Alto with Bill, a fellow classics major, and his friend Rick, a junior at Stanford who also hoped to be a doctor. After suffering some sort of breakdown, the cause of which remained a mystery to me, Bill moved out after less than a month, which left Rick and me in need of another housemate to help pay the rent. I convinced my friend Gene to take the third bedroom.

Neal, who dropped by the house periodically, nicknamed Rick, who was half Mexican and half Swiss, Li'l Rick because of his short stature and boyish looks, but Rick comported himself like a man much older. A stutter made him cautious and introspective. When he was about to speak, he'd flutter his eyes as he gathered his thoughts; and when the words finally emerged, he spoke in a precise, melodious baritone that I found charming. As the weeks passed, Rick often made provocative remarks. When I told him that I planned to travel to Europe the following summer before medical school, he asked with a mischievous smile, "Oh, are you going to go to *Gay* Par-ee?" On another occasion he wondered if I knew anything about glory holes. When I later learned that a glory hole was an aperture in a bathroom stall through which you could stick your erect penis and get a blowjob, I blushed with embarrassment. *Blowjob* wasn't a term I was familiar with either, and I'd never had or given one. The idea of a glory hole disgusted me, not so much the blowjob but its place in an unsanitary public restroom. I found myself puzzling over Rick's motives.

One fall evening in 1976, the three of us celebrated Gene's acceptance into a graduate program in Slavic languages. Gene let us know that the Russian way to celebrate was to chase down black bread with shots of vodka. He'd procured some cheap vodka, but we had only a loaf of stale pumpernickel, so we sat around the kitchen table washing down chunks of terrible bread with the bitter clear liquid. It didn't take much to get us drunk. Then Rick vomited in the bushes outside the front door, which prompted Gene, who was highly suggestible, to vomit before he fell asleep clutching the toilet bowl. As I nursed Rick on the sofa, we began to touch each other affectionately. In the heat of the moment, shirts were unbuttoned and pants unzipped. We weren't naked, but Gene would have been shocked had he somehow arisen and stumbled onto us. What struck me later was how natural sex with a man was for me, even though it was my first experience. Rick remarked that he'd never kissed anyone with a beard before.

As our relationship progressed, Rick began to express doubts about being gay. I wrote to him a number of times from Europe, but his responses were full of ambivalence. Before I started classes at Northwestern at the end of September 1977, he traveled to Chicago for his own interview at the medical school. I was staying with my parents briefly until I could move into my dormitory room on campus, and he stayed in their guest room. Despite an overwhelming sexual attraction to him, I didn't dare linger too long with him. I'd said nothing to my parents about our relationship and wasn't prepared to deal with such a revelation at this point in my life, when I didn't yet have a full gay identity. Afterward I took a Greyhound bus with Rick back to San Francisco, holding his hand under a blanket throughout the forty-eight-hour ride across the dull midsection of the United States. But then we argued about our feelings for each other and parted abruptly. On the bus ride back to Chicago I slept fitfully and read four novels by John Steinbeck, an author who'd attended Stanford—my way of keeping a connection to the university I revered and had parted from sadly—as a way to push Rick out of my mind.

Early in the first quarter, I hung out with a classmate named Mark. At 6:30 in the morning he would knock on my door in Abbott Hall to join him for a run on a nearby track or to play racquetball. In high school I'd had no interest in sports. I refused to learn to swim, I detested wrestling, and the most I was willing to do in gymnastics was a somersault. Sweating disgusted me, and group showering, which would have been a kind of heaven for most gay boys, intimidated me, in part because I didn't reach puberty until the age of sixteen and felt more shame about my own childish body parts than curiosity about the mature body parts of others. When I went to college, I was a five-foot-eight-and-a-half-inch narrow-shouldered adolescent who weighed 120 pounds. In California, land of the bronzed six-packs, I made a concerted effort to improve my physique and took up weightlifting. In one year I gained twenty-five pounds. I also developed a passion for long-distance running. The Stanford campus sprawled across nine thousand acres, much of it undeveloped and wonderful to explore. In Chicago I looked for another way to exercise, especially in the winter, when only the obsessed ran outdoors. Mark introduced me to squash and racquetball, sports I turned out to have an aptitude for.

In the first three months of medical school, Mark and I spent so much time together that others noticed. He introduced me to opera, and we attended chamber music and vocal recitals performed by his numerous musician friends. Once when he invited me to the symphony while we were in the dorm cafeteria, a female classmate asked with amusement, "Is that a date?" Although the question sailed passed him, I was mortified. By the end of December I was infatuated with Mark. We'd just finished playing racquetball one evening—unusual because typically we played in the morning, but that day my job drawing blood at the VA hospital interfered with our daily ritual—and as he reclined on his bed bare-chested, rather provocatively, I thought, I declared my feelings for him.

I wasn't prepared for his reaction. Flushed and confused, he squirmed into a shirt and demanded that I leave. My apologies fell flat. For the rest of the academic year he avoided me, and the following fall he transferred to a medical school in New York City, explaining to classmates that he wanted to be closer to his parents' home on the East Coast. It may have been the truth, but I was deeply hurt.

During orientation to medical school, when various individuals or organizations were allowed to make presentations to the incoming class, one courageous soul, a second-year student named Eric, invited any of us who might be gay to contact him about forming a gay medical student group. The general response was polite startlement; no one stirred. At the time it didn't strike me how remarkable it was that he'd been permitted to raise what I considered to be, in retrospect, a taboo subject; a more conservative administration might have blocked him. I didn't approach Eric until the spring of 1978, after I'd recovered from Mark's rebuff. Although I got on well with all 160 members of my class, I felt lonely and isolated. I had my confidants—Neal and my high school friend Doug—but they lived elsewhere. A number of classmates had paired up, and others were married or engaged. I knew that there had to be a handful of others like me—and I had my suspicions—but all of us lacked Eric's courage. Rather than congregating, we behaved like poles of a magnet and sat far from each other even during classes.

Eric introduced me to Chicago's gay bar scene. After we went out one night, he seduced me, and we had sex in his room at Abbott Hall. As we made out on the cold floor, I tried to drum up enthusiasm for him, but it wasn't sex I'd been looking for; I was looking for friendship. I later resented the quid pro quo nature of our relationship—as a reward for being my guide, he expected me to have sex with him. I was still too green to understand the casual nature of sex for many gay men. For me, sex was the consummation of a relationship, not the initiation of one. But perhaps I wasn't as different from other gay men, or men in general, as I thought. While struggling to satisfy Eric's needs that night, I noted his flaccid pecs and hairy paunch, a combination of features that repelled me. Perhaps if he'd had a beefier physique and handsomer face, I'd have gladly given up my Victorian views.

I spent much of the summer in search of love but had to settle for a few unsatisfying hookups. One September evening at Alfie's, my gaze landed on Art. He squeezed his way toward me and offered to buy me a beer. Short, balding, and muscular, he had a thick brown mustache, a warm smile, and dazzling blue eyes. He wore a T-shirt, cowboy boots, and tight jeans that bunched up suggestively at his crotch, the stereotype of a butch gay man in the late 1970s. Although I didn't find him good-looking, I felt an animal attraction to him. His face lit up when I told him that I was a medical student. He was in the healthcare business too, he said. He embraced me, which made me uncomfortable because the gesture was unexpected and presumptuous, but I was also excited and flattered.

Fourteen years older than I, Art was an ordained minister and executive director of a retirement facility in the suburbs, which explained his winning way with people and why I felt at ease with him after just a few minutes. He told me that he had been born on the West Coast, grew up on a farm, and attended seminary in New York City before relocating to the Chicago area after spending time in New Orleans as a pastor in a church. He'd married and had two young daughters, but his wife filed for divorce when she discovered that he was having sex with men. His move to the city from the suburbs had been abrupt; he brought with him only his clothes, his car, and a few possessions.

Art took me to his apartment, a dismal place on the edge of Uptown in a type of building called a four-plus-one, a cheap brick and glass midrise with paper-thin walls. Inside you could hear car doors banging and the dumpster top slam shut as if they were in the room next door. His place was furnished with a teak table and chairs in the living room, but we went quickly to the large bed in the bedroom, which overlooked an uninspiring courtyard. After sex, we fell asleep. The next morning he projected a different persona, reserved and businesslike. I watched him in the mirror as he dressed in a three-piece suit, strength, ambition, and resolve in his eyes. He apologized for not driving me back to my apartment because he was heading in the opposite direction, but we exchanged numbers and promised to get together again. I'd enjoyed the night and felt sad at our parting. I'd used to smirk at the speed at which young couples fell in love in operas after one or two arias, like Rudolfo and Mimi in *La Boheme* or Alfredo and Violetta in *La Traviata*, but great composers hit on a simple truth: we attach ourselves quickly to the objects of our desire. After one night, I was attached.

The next night Art called me, and we met again two days later. In his apartment was another young man named Jim. Exceptionally lean, perhaps ill (in medical terminology I would have referred to him as cachectic), he had a handlebar mustache and mischievous green eyes. Jim stayed there while Art and I went to dinner and was gone when we returned. A year later Art told me that he had told Jim about his latest trick, and that Jim had dared him to call me so he could size me up. I surprised him when I appeared at the door, because I wasn't the person he'd imagined, although I didn't disappoint him. He claimed that he'd been drunk the night we met and suffered from a hangover the next morning. I'm not sure why Art told me this; I didn't think it was funny, if humor was the intent. Jim's presence that night turned out to be an omen, in more ways than one.

In the beginning, Art seemed to have all the ingredients I'd been searching for: maturity, stability, and keen intelligence. I viewed the age difference as an asset, not a liability. At twenty-four, not yet fully comfortable in my gay skin and uncertain of my future, I looked to him for guidance. It wasn't just his age; it was his position in life. Even as an unbeliever, I held clergymen in as high regard as I did doctors, viewing them as two-dimensional heroes rather than complex human beings with contradictions and character flaws. Most alluring to me, Art took an almost childish delight in what the world had to offer. He enjoyed fine dining, tolerated opera, and accompanied me to marathon films like *Shoah*, a nine-hour French documentary that investigated the origins of the Holocaust, and *Napoleon*, a silent movie accompanied by live music from the Chicago Symphony Orchestra. He also had a penchant for travel. We spent our second Christmas together in Paris, the most romantic city in the world, and another week in Florence. Later we traveled farther afield to East Africa, Israel, and the Sinai Desert.

But Art also caused me a great deal of grief. During the first year of our relationship, he gave me three sexually transmitted infections: crab lice, gonorrhea, and hepatitis B. His infidelities and their health consequences led to numerous arguments and promises from him to be faithful. Had I been a stronger person, I'd have bolted. Instead I rationalized everything, believing that I could transform him into a monogamous partner by laying down ground rules that in the end only I would follow. And in fact he'd acquired the gonorrhea he gave me from an old boyfriend, who'd spent several days with him while I sulked at home over another betrayal.

After that first year, I never developed another venereal disease. When he discovered a cluster of anal warts, I wasn't too concerned because they could have predated me in his life. I accompanied him several times to the office of a surgeon, one of the few at the time who treated venereal warts in gay men. The topical treatment was painful and curtailed our sexual activity, which had already dwindled, although not entirely for altruistic reasons. Art traveled a lot, or so he said. Sometimes he would be gone for weeks at a time, or he canceled a planned weekend together at the last minute because he had to go out of town or spend time with his daughters. As a trade-off for less sex, he mollified me with expressions of deep affection, which allowed him to carry on a carefully choreographed deception that took me years to discover. I believe he enjoyed spending time with me—perhaps he even loved me—but his compulsion for sex with multiple partners created a conflict that he didn't know how to resolve.

My love for Art was both hidden from the world and obsessive. Early in our relationship I was devoted to him. It was the reverse of poor Albertine in Proust's *In Search of Lost Time*, whom the jealous narrator holds as a near prisoner in order to keep her away from other potential lovers. In my case, I was my own captor. In theory, a captive can escape a captor, but I couldn't escape myself. *What a life!* I later thought. As the years passed, I spent many evenings sitting by the telephone waiting for his call, and canceling plans with other friends at the last minute when he did finally phone. I even failed to attend the wedding of one of my medical school friends because I worried about what Art might be doing in my absence. I lied to my parents about why I couldn't come to their home for dinner on a Saturday night. My excuses were lame and unconvincing. They were worse than the truth, because I was dishonest; but the truth seemed worse to me than any excuse I could drum up.

Although I socialized with my classmates before and after lectures, during labs, and later on our clinical rotations, at night I escaped to a different world. I still found time to study, and during my clerkships, when medical students spent four weeks on each of the primary care services like internal medicine, psychiatry, pediatrics, obstetrics-gynecology, and general surgery, I never missed a day or night of call. But I made no room in my life for anyone except Art, which meant lonely nights when he wasn't around. I experienced great emotional extremes: elation when we were together, profound sadness and frustration when we were apart. At the same time, shame ruled me: shame for betraying my friends and family, shame for being gay, shame for my dependence on someone who would never fully commit himself to me, each manifestation of shame playing off the others.

Not my family, my friends, or the marvels of the city but Art bound me to Chicago. If you'd asked me in 1977 where I'd be after medical school, I'd have declared Northern California, where I longed to stroll along rugged seascapes or hike majestic mountains or bike through rolling foothills burnished a velvety brown in the autumn sun. But because of his daughters Art couldn't leave Chicago, and despite the impossibility of ever feeling fulfilled in this relationship, I was too attached to him to consider moving somewhere else. It was an old story, a timeless story, even a cliché, and the central subject of many novels, films, operas, Broadway musicals, and contemporary love songs. The only difference was that for me, trapped by shame and fear of the world's wrath—some of it genuine, some of it imaginary—my love for another man was still a love that dared not speak its name.

: 4 :

Art's Final Illness

(1985)

Over the span of our relationship, from September 1978 to April 1983, Art often complained about his health. Sometimes it was a sore throat or stiff neck. He'd open his mouth for me to peer in or ask me to put a hand to his forehead to check for a fever. In the early days I found this endearing, and it was a good opportunity to practice on a live patient. Most of the time he had nothing more than a cold; an ordinary muscle spasm caused the stiff neck. He was self-conscious about his fingers and toes, which were gnarled with arthritis, a result of manual labor as a child on his grandparents' farm in the Northwest. Nothing could be done about those deformities. His bowel problems often amused me because I knew they weren't due to anything serious. Wincing with pain from an abdominal cramp, he'd dash to the bathroom and then emerge to report—perhaps because I was training to be a doctor; otherwise why would I care—that he'd only expelled gas. Once, after drinking too much sangria in Spain, he lost control of his bowels before reaching our hotel. *So typical*, I thought, without daring to laugh because to him, shit streaming down his pant leg, it was no laughing matter. Except for that embarrassing incident, I attributed his various maladies and complaints to stress, anxiety, or neurosis.

But then more severe illnesses afflicted him. In 1980 he wound up in the hospital on intravenous antibiotics after a pimple he squeezed in his mustache became infected. Within twenty-four hours the lower part of his face and upper lip ballooned. I sat next to his bed, held his hand, and watched bad TV with him, assuring him that he'd soon be better. In 1981 he developed necrotizing gingivitis, a nasty, foul-smelling gum infection that required antibiotics and multiple painful procedures to debride the inflamed tissues. In early 1983 he broke out in shingles. A thick band of blisters, pustules, and scabs extended from his right lower back around to his lower abdomen, into his groin, and down his right leg. For weeks he writhed in agony and lived on narcotic pain relievers.

Facial cellulitis, gingivitis, or shingles can afflict anyone during his lifetime. Individually, each disease usually has no clinical significance, as we say. Collectively, however, they pointed to something abnormal with Art's immune system. I didn't think of it that way then; I just thought he was suffering from bad luck.

But that was in 1983, when we were still a couple, albeit a fraught and doomed one. When he came into the office in mid-June 1985, I became alarmed. In only one month he'd lost twenty pounds. His pants were pulled up and secured above his waist, in the manner of someone twice his age. He might have looked buffoonish, but there wasn't anything funny about his appearance. It was clear to me that he was deathly ill, although it wasn't clear to me that he knew it. Tom put him in the hospital for a full evaluation.

That day, recalling all those illnesses, and the sexually transmitted diseases I'd contracted from him, brought my life to a sudden halt. My heart raced, sweat streamed down the side of my face and stained my armpits, and I wanted to vomit. My general health was excellent, but everyone with AIDS felt well until a cough evolved into a life-threatening pneumonia, hazy vision progressed to irreversible blindness, or loose stools transformed into a cholera-like dysentery. I didn't know for sure that Art had AIDS. He could have had some sort of cancer. But given his age of forty-five, there were few other diseases that could explain his debilitated condition.

I had first read about AIDS in July or August 1981 in the library of St. Joe's, not long after starting my internship. I often hung out there when I had nothing to do or while I waited for notification of another admission. Among the journals there was an unfamiliar one about the size of *Reader's Digest* called *The Morbidity and Mortality Weekly Report*, or *MMWR*, published by the Centers for Disease Control in Atlanta. I picked up the June 5 issue because of an article, "Dengue Type 4 Infections in U.S. Travelers to the Caribbean." Sometimes I fantasized about traipsing through Central Africa or some other exotic locale, as a medical sleuth tracking down tropical or subtropical diseases with unusual names like leishmaniasis and dranunculiasis.

In my habitual scrubs and a long blue lab coat, I headed to a table and opened the journal, my stethoscope and other instruments clattering in my pockets as I sat down. I was stunned by the lead article, which described five previously healthy homosexual men in Los Angeles who'd been diagnosed with pneumocystis pneumonia (PCP) between October 1980 and May 1981. Eventually four of the five young men had died—which was remarkable since at that time only premature or malnourished infants with underdeveloped immune systems or older children and adults on chemotherapy developed life-threatening infections from PCP. They had some sort of unidentified disease—one with no name yet.

I read more issues of *MMWR*. In the July 3 issue the CDC described an "outbreak" of Kaposi's sarcoma (KS) in gay men in New York City as well as California, but KS was a type of cancer arising from the lining of blood vessels, not an infection, or so we thought at the time. Were these diseases something I as a gay man in Chicago was supposed to worry about? As a young doctor, would I ever see a case?

I vaguely recalled having read about PCP in a textbook during medical school, but I had paid little attention to it. I knew something of KS, which I'd encountered in the dermatology clinic at the VA hospital in an elderly man who had purplish nodules on his lower legs. I was lucky to see one, the dermatology resident told me; she'd seen only one other case. It was an indolent disease with no treatment; the man would probably die of something else.

We called conditions like PCP and KS "zebras" because of their rarity. There's an adage in medicine: "When you hear hoofbeats, think of horses, not zebras." Once in medical school, a lecturer led off by flashing a slide of a herd of zebras on the African plains. If someone has a headache, he said, the most likely cause is a muscle spasm, not a brain tumor. An otherwise healthy patient with a cough, fever, shortness of breath, and an abnormal chest x-ray probably has pneumonia caused by a common organism, easily treated with an antibiotic. In our differential diagnosis, as we called the list of possible causes of an ailment, we should rule out common problems first before wasting time and money looking for something obscure. We couldn't know then that the obscure would become common, turning the aphorism on its head.

Soon other strange infections in previously healthy gay men were noted. Three men died of complications from herpes simplex. In most people, herpes is an annoying cluster of blisters and scabs on the lips, penis, anus, or vulva that heal without any treatment; but in these three men, herpes went wild, invading internal organs and the brain. Cytomegalovirus (CMV) blinded two other men. Baffled and worried that these cases were just the tip of an iceberg, the CDC established a task force to search for cases elsewhere in the country and conduct laboratory investigations to unearth a cause. By the end of the year, the CDC had documented seventy-three cases of KS in men under the age of fifty, an unheard-of number. Before 1979 public health officials hadn't noticed an uptick in cases of KS in the cancer registry, and KS continued to occur in its usual demographic population, men of Ashkenazi Jewish or Mediterranean heritage older than sixty years of age. Beginning in 1981, the number climbed exponentially.

For obvious reasons, the disease piqued my interest. Whenever an article popped up describing more cases or speculating on a possible cause, I filed it away, but at first there wasn't much published in the medical literature. The *New York Times, San Francisco Chronicle,* and other coastal papers followed the story, but elsewhere the disease wasn't on the radar. Then, in December 1981, the *Lancet,* a respected British medical journal, published a two-page article titled "Immunocompromised Homosexuals." With its juxtaposition of two negative words, the title struck me as judgmen-

tal. It was bad enough to be a homosexual in 1981. Now a pejora-
tive adjective made the noun seem worse than ever. As I read the
article, I underlined critical points as if I were preparing for an examination—or my potential obituary. "The case fatality rate ... has
been an alarming 40 %," the authors wrote. "As well as their sexual
preference, almost all of the patients have had in common ... evidence of infection with CMV. ... Some other factors, acting alone
or together with CMV, must be responsible for the depression of
... immunity." Another *Lancet* article in February 1982 suggested a
connection between the regular use of amyl or butyl nitrite, commonly known as "poppers," an inhaled stimulant that enhances
sexual arousal, and the development of opportunistic infections.
In some circles the disease came to be known as GRID: gay-related-
immune-deficiency disorder.

One of those circles was Howard Brown, where we volunteer
doctors spoke to each other tersely between patients about this
potential threat to our community. It was easy to dismiss the reports
as curiosities, limited mainly to New York and California. Typical
epidemics, like influenza, cholera, or the plague, sweep quickly
through populations. Other infectious diseases, like meningitis in
soldiers' barracks or college dormitories, wreak havoc on a small
number of people before burning out. Would this disease become
a true epidemic, or would it burn out? We had no idea. In Chicago
we weren't freaked out yet, just wary.

It wasn't long before GRID appeared in other US cities. I saw my
first case in the fall of 1982, during a rotation in the intensive care
unit. The unfortunate patient was a young gay man with PCP, the
second case identified in Illinois. His primary physician was Tom.
By the time he came to the ICU, he was on a ventilator, his lungs so
congested that he couldn't oxygenate his blood and needed artificial assistance to stay alive. His body was riddled with KS, purplish
tumors of various shapes and sizes appearing on his face, trunk,
and arms. Some looked like bruises, as if he'd been beaten up. I was
as horrified as I was fascinated not only by the ugly eruptions on his
body but also because everything we tried to do to save him failed.

He was an anonymous patient, like so many who wound up in

the ICU who couldn't speak because of a tube shoved into their lungs and whose lives were snuffed out before we even knew their names. I knew nothing about his life, loves, or work, which would have transformed him from a helpless object in a hospital bed into a three-dimensional human being. There was no one at his bedside or sitting anxiously in the waiting area, no boyfriend, parent, or sibling to fill in the blanks of his life, to help us understand how this might have happened. I couldn't feel his fear because, thankfully, he was heavily sedated. And of course I had no idea that he was a harbinger of terrible things to come.

Because we didn't know how he'd acquired this disease, we donned caps, gowns, gloves, and booties and covered our mouths with surgical masks and eyes with goggles. Dr. B., the thoracic surgeon who'd opened the patient's chest to obtain a lung biopsy, which ultimately provided us with enough tissue to make the PCP diagnosis, tore off the protective armor and proclaimed in a stentorian voice that the patient wasn't contagious. Because we trusted him, we cast off our masks too. It was like removing a helmet in space and finding that you could breathe.

I saw a different form of the disease in my clinic in late 1982. On the recommendation of the staff of Howard Brown, which would become a significant referral source for my growing practice, a young man came in with enlarged lymph nodes. Knots were visible in the back of his neck. I felt rubbery lumps under his armpits and in his groin. He had no other symptoms and looked perfectly healthy. Most people who developed generalized lymphadenopathy, as he had, eventually sickened with full-blown AIDS, but we didn't know that yet.

By this time the disease was popping up in populations besides gay men. What connected these cases mystified everyone, including my friends at Howard Brown and me. We debated possible links—genetic, environmental, or infectious. The threat was both vague and palpable because we didn't know who among us was truly at risk, though people in four distinct and seemingly unrelated groups—the four Hs: homosexuals, heroin addicts, Haitians, and hemophiliacs—were getting sick and dying. There was a colossal storm out there, but we couldn't figure out when or where it would strike.

As a result, we had no idea how to counsel our patients or protect ourselves. No one wanted to admit that AIDS was transmitted through sex. The closest example of a disease that was both sexually transmitted and blood-borne was hepatitis B. A good number of men did show up at Howard Brown with yellow eyes and ghastly yellow skin. They complained of nausea, urine as dark as Earl Grey tea, and shit the color of clay. I could assure most of them that they'd be fine. In fact, more than two-thirds of gay men in that era tested positive for exposure to hepatitis B. I was one of them, thanks to Art. Before the Red Cross began screening blood donations for it, you could acquire hepatitis B through a blood transfusion. Although 10 percent of people with hepatitis B developed chronic infections, only a fraction of those progressed to cirrhosis of the liver or liver cancer. Otherwise it was rarely fatal. No one wanted it, but hepatitis B didn't terrify us. And it didn't change our sexual behavior.

But as new cases of AIDS were reported nationwide, public health officials urged gay men everywhere to start using condoms, even when having oral sex. Epidemiologists surmised that AIDS was some sort of infectious disease, definitely blood borne and possibly carried in other bodily fluids. To many men, using a condom for a blowjob seemed unappetizing and unromantic. Some officials went further and advocated that gay men abstain from all forms of sex until further notice, a recommendation that provoked an outcry in the gay community. After struggling so hard to gain acceptance, gay men were being told to give up what they'd been fighting for, the freedom to love whom they desired. Hadn't many straight people ignored religious dictates to abstain from sex until after marriage?

I wish that I'd been the Paul Revere of the Chicago gay community. I wasn't. Despite the surge in cases reported nationwide, there were still fewer than two thousand at the end of 1982 and only a handful of them were in Illinois, a number that didn't impress me. Lacking a firm grounding in the mathematics of epidemics, I wasn't as alarmed as I should have been, especially since it hadn't been absolutely proved that the cause was infectious. The virus that caused it wasn't identified for more than another year. And at this time Art and I were still together, and we were still, infrequently, having sex. Like many other young gay men, I remained in a state of denial about my risk.

In 1984, scientists in the United States and France announced that a virus caused AIDS. That virus, called both LAV for lymphadenopathy-associated virus and HTLV-III for human T-lymphocyte virus III, had the perverse ability to take control of a cell and turn it into a factory that made more viruses, which in turn would infect other cells. You could find the virus in semen, vaginal secretions, rectal tissue, and blood and blood products, which explained the connection between the four major groups of people afflicted at that time. Because of competing claims of discovery of the causative agent—was it found by Luc Montagnier, a French scientist, or Robert Gallo, an American scientist?—for a couple of years the virus bore the unwieldy name HTLV-III/LAV. It was later renamed the human immunodeficiency virus: HIV.

In the summer of 1985, when Art came to the clinic in such bad shape, there was still no way to know with absolute certainty if a person had been infected by the AIDS virus, because a test for it wasn't commercially available, although research laboratories and the American Red Cross, which controlled the nation's blood supply, were already using an unlicensed test. You made the diagnosis of AIDS when someone presented with some horrific infection caused by organisms, ordinarily harmless, that are given the opportunity to wreak havoc when the person's immune system loses its ability to protect them: hence the term opportunistic infection. Until the advent of chemotherapy and AIDS, we had no idea we were such a complex ecosystem, full of microbes kept in check and balance by a highly efficient and hypervigilant immune system. During childhood we are exposed to many of these microbes—viruses, bacteria, and fungi—that at worst cause a brief illness, are subdued, and then hide like sleeper cells, waiting for a call to action that usually never comes in a normal life. But once that checks-and-balances system is disrupted, it's as if the prison guards (in this case, so-called T helper cells and a type of white blood cell called a macrophage) have been killed and the dangerous criminals inside the prison set free.

Although the natural history of AIDS, the time period from onset of infection to overt disease, hadn't been worked out by 1985, I had to wonder if Art had harbored the virus for some time before we broke up in April 1983. The implication of that for me was obvious.

Our final split had been long in coming. One Sunday afternoon in late February 1983, on the way home from the hospital—I was now living just a few blocks from my old haunts, Northwestern Medical Center and Alfie's—I ran into Art, who was carrying a newly purchased record under his right arm and walking with a handsome man who was around thirty years old, like me. I was surprised because Art had told me he was spending the weekend with his daughters. After he introduced me to Max, I hurried on and didn't look back.

My chest felt heavy, as if I'd swallowed a lead weight. A year earlier I would have been shattered, but Art's long absences had eventually made me more independent. I spent a good deal of my free time reading novels, hanging out with new friends, and playing the piano. I was happy as a family practice resident, caring for patients and making difficult decisions that could have positive impacts on people's lives; and I enjoyed volunteering at Howard Brown, counseling gay men and treating their venereal diseases. But now I felt sad and angry. Since we saw each other so infrequently because of his travels, I was offended that Art dared to spend his free time with another man in Chicago. If I'd been in Art's place, he would have been the first person I called after I stepped off the airplane.

I stopped at the grocery store and picked up a few items. My head swam as if I'd just awakened from a deep sleep. As soon as I entered my apartment and took off my coat, I went to the bathroom to look in the mirror. I wasn't displeased with what I saw. In fact, I thought I looked rather good, except for a few wisps of hair that crossed my forehead. I brushed them back and turned my head from side to side, trying to be objective about my appearance. My face didn't glisten as it had when I was younger, and I had no embarrassing pimples. I flashed a smile of white, well-aligned teeth. It occurred to me that I was measuring myself against Max, little as I knew about his relationship with Art or what he knew of my own. I had the unpleasant notion that my battle might have been one-sided—Art could easily have passed me off as a doctor friend. "We're heading up north," Max had said, not realizing how insolent those words sounded to me, implying he and Art were a couple. And perhaps they were.

Several days passed before Art called me. The first thing he said was that he couldn't talk long. My heart paused for a moment before pounding wildly. I still yearned for love, a fulfilling sex life, and a lasting relationship with another man. But I knew that Art was going to tell me something I didn't want to hear.

Max was going to move in with him and occupy the second bedroom. This news surprised me. Art had always refused to share an apartment with me because of his daughters and the reaction of his ex-wife, who might sue him for exclusive custody. I'd accepted that excuse and even considered it wise. Now it was clear that he'd had other reasons for keeping me distant. Too angry for tears, I restrained myself from slamming down the receiver and shattering it.

———

Two years later, on the night of his hospital admission to St. Joe's, I telephoned Art there, but the operator informed me that "this particular patient" had requested anonymity. His name hadn't been entered in the computer, and he wasn't accepting phone calls. His request struck me as yet another example of the complex web of deception he wove around his life.

I decided to visit Art the following day. I hoped to put a period at the end of the sentence, to end a chapter in my life. He had once been the primary object of my affection and had consumed so much of my waking life, and I had so many questions for him, some philosophical, others crude, but none professional: when did you fall out of love with me; could I have done something to save the relationship; how many men did you fuck when we were together; how many fucked you? Although I realized that the answers to such questions can become unimportant in an emotional if not medical sense, not enough time had passed for me to cease yearning for some sort of closure. The breakup still stung.

But when I walked into Art's room dressed in my long gray medical frock, I didn't have the heart to confront him. He was in good spirits and overjoyed to see me. Except for his weight loss, he looked surprisingly well. Hydration had filled out his sunken cheeks; his eyes sparkled with life. I sat on the edge of his bed and talked to him for fifteen minutes or so, resisting the temptation to review our joint history because it was his health that mattered now, not my selfish needs. He asked me if I thought he had "the Big One," meaning AIDS. I didn't know, I answered in a professional monotone. No test results were back. Then he said that he'd "really cut back" on his sexual activity and had "done nothing" for two years. He said he was on the verge of working out a huge deal in Louisiana that had preoccupied him for seven or eight years, and he couldn't believe that now he was sick.

"I guess I'll have to let them know the full story, if I do have AIDS," he said nonchalantly, a remark that struck me as bold since I presumed he was still in the closet at work.

At once a surge of irritation filled me as I thought about all those times I sat alone waiting for his call when in fact he was having sex with other men. Those extended travels to cities across the country on business had been a ruse. I doubted that he had a huge deal in Louisiana, or anywhere for that matter. Maintaining my composure, I said nothing.

A few months before our breakup, I had passed by his apartment on the way home from Seton. He had moved to a Gold Coast address, a ten-minute walk from mine, that was tonier and more appropriate for an executive director of a healthcare facility than that roach-infested apartment on the edge of Uptown. When I noticed the glow of light from his living room that evening, I was surprised and delighted. Assuming he'd returned to Chicago earlier than expected from one of his out-of-town jaunts, I went over.

The doorman, a friendly but formal man who knew me well, let me in without calling Art first, and I took the elevator to the fourteenth floor. When I knocked on Art's door, no one answered. After knocking harder, I heard a commotion and a thud of approaching footsteps. Cracking the door open, Art blushed with embarrassment and expressed annoyance at my unsolicited appearance. He was half-dressed and disheveled, but not in the manner of someone who'd fallen asleep on the couch after a hard day's work or long hours in airports. Through the crack I glimpsed other men who scurried out of sight and laughed as Art waved them off. I also sniffed the skunky odor of marijuana.

Without waiting for an excuse or an apology, I backtracked to the elevator on the verge of tears and rushed out of the building past the doorman, who made no comment but, like all doormen, understood more about the human condition than most people. Feeling shocked, humiliated, and angry, I knew that I could never face that doorman again. And yet despite all the evidence to the contrary, I still believed that somehow I could salvage my relationship with Art.

The blinders lifted after our breakup. Friends filled in the details afterward, confessing that they never had the heart to tell me what they knew—the sex parties in Chicago and other cities, the frequent tricks he brought home—because I wouldn't have believed them. But they were right about my degree of denial.

Now, in the hospital, Art made no references to past escapades or their effect on me, and I didn't press him. It was difficult for me to remember all the wonderful times we'd spent together—the intimate moments in his apartment (although not once in four and a half years did he spend a night in my apartment), the operas, plays, and concerts we attended, the dinners in trendy restaurants, and our travels. It was the negatives that had thrown us back together.

The conversation remained lighthearted, with only brief references to weightier issues, but I felt burdened. I looked around the cramped room with its ugly furnishings—the cheap tray table with its half-empty cup of tea and dirty napkins, the metal cabinet with faux plywood finish, the clunky hospital bed. All were illuminated by the glaring fluorescent light above the headboard. The awkward feeling was mine, not his, as if I were the patient under examination and he the doctor impassively observing my idiosyncrasies and imperfections.

The following day a clerk from Cook County Hospital called our office with the results of Art's stool specimen. In 1985 the microbiologists at St. Joe's weren't adept at identifying uncommon parasites; if they suspected something unusual, they sent the specimen for a second opinion from Cook County, whose pathology department was among the best in the country. County's expertise arose from its clientele—including immigrants, criminals, substance abusers, and the indigent who flocked in the thousands every year for medical care not otherwise available to them. Its emergency department was the medical equivalent of a bazaar, where you could find anything from the mundane like the common cold to the violent like gunshot wounds and fearsome injuries from stabbings, to the locally rare like malaria.

Tom and I happened to emerge from our exam rooms almost simultaneously when Art's result was posted. We both looked at the pink message slip: "positive cryptosporidium," which our receptionist had recorded with dispassionate simplicity. In healthy people, cryptosporidium causes an annoying case of diarrhea that can last a few days or weeks without serious harm. In someone with an impaired immune system, the results are catastrophic. In Art's case, it meant he had AIDS.

Years earlier I had been in a bicycle accident, catapulting over the handlebars at high speed and tumbling head over heels to the ground. The flight seemed to occur in slow motion, as if I were watching it happen to someone else. When I got up, I was in shock. I checked to see if I was still whole and noticed that a triangle of flesh had been sliced off my left wrist. Then my heart pounded, the wound burned, and I was overwhelmed with fear: oh my God, I could have broken a bone, been paralyzed from the neck down, or died! But I was alive; only the bicycle was mangled.

I was in that slow-motion flight again now. Tom thought I was going to faint. All the blood had drained from my face, and my mouth felt parched. Tom extended a hand, but I didn't take it. My brain raced a trillion miles away to some black hole before returning to earth. I gripped the back of a chair and trembled, as if the temperature had dropped 30 degrees. Art had just been given a death sentence, and I believed I'd gotten one too. I spent the rest of the day performing my professional functions in a fog, going through the motions of interviewing and examining people but not paying attention to their symptoms or physical findings.

I didn't know how to present the news to Gavin, my boyfriend, when I returned to the apartment we shared in the Old Town neighborhood. I usually didn't walk down North Avenue at night—the darkened recesses of its dilapidated buildings were too disturbing—but I was so absorbed in thought that I forgot my usual fears. With the awful task uppermost in my mind, I would have gladly surrendered to some mugger without a fight.

After dating for more than a year, Gavin and I had moved in together just two months earlier. Although marriage wasn't possible, cohabitation was close. When I informed my parents about the move, it was under the guise that Gavin and I were roommates, two young doctors splitting expenses, something matter-of-fact and of no other significance. I'd never told them anything about Art, whose presence in my life would have been hard to explain without lying.

Although my father seemed to have no clue about the true nature of my relationship with Gavin, my mother had her suspicions. As they visited the duplex apartment one Sunday afternoon, I heard her shushing my father when he wondered aloud about the absence of a second bedroom. Gavin and I glanced at each other in silence, but I let an opportunity to have a heart-to-heart discussion with my parents slip by.

Before meeting Gavin—and based on my experience with Art and many novels—*Anna Karenina, Madame Bovary, In Search of Lost Time*—I had concluded that suffering was an integral part of a forbidden relationship, perhaps the essential part. I also believed that relationships were lopsided, with one person always more attached than the other. In my limited experience, gay men seemed to prize infidelity over monogamy, hoping to fuck as many men as possible. Stroll down Halsted Street on any Saturday night, enter a bar, and observe the throngs of men, some packed into dark corners giving or getting blowjobs; or notice the men streaming in and out of a popular bathhouse, a place I knew all about but had never set foot in. I didn't need that sort of affirmation; and I didn't have that kind of sexual appetite. All I wanted was a "normal" relationship, like that of any heterosexual couple.

Gavin had moved to Chicago in June 1983 before starting his residency at St. Joe's. I'd interviewed him the previous October and given him my card, but thought nothing more about him until he sent me a letter in May, asking if he could stay with me for a few days while looking for an apartment. It was an unusual request, but I consented. Art and I had broken up, and I was single and alone. That first night, a bare-chested Gavin slipped into a sleeping bag on the living-room floor, propping himself up on his elbows and casting coy glances at me as we talked about the training program, the medical staff, and other matters related to his future. The next morning I took him to breakfast at Ann Sather's, the gayest restaurant in Chicago at the time, but he said nothing about the clientele. As we walked through Boys' Town, the heart of gay life in Chicago, in search of apartments, he ignored the gay bars we passed. I felt foolish and wondered if I'd misinterpreted his cues.

After he left, I had wild, disturbing thoughts about him prompted by seeing *Querelle*, a violent homoerotic film by the gay German filmmaker Rainer Werner Fassbinder. It was a daring film, one of the first to advance gay themes, a must-see for a gay man. Photographed in a gauzy light, it felt more like a hallucination to me than a coherent movie, its action shifting from a ship to a bar with male and female whores, to a urinal and later a prison cell. The men lusted after each other yet threatened to murder each other, love and death (or Eros and Thanatos as in Greek mythology), vying for domination. At one point Querelle, a sailor more beautiful than handsome, performed a stylized dance with his brother, each man clutching a jackknife in his fist at groin level, left foot crossing right foot in an ever-tightening circle like the gang members facing off in *West Side Story*. I exited the theater with my heart pounding and my throat constricted with anguish. My erotic feelings for Art had not yet been extinguished, and now they were transferred to Gavin, which made me feel ashamed because my gay-dar might have misled me. Months later, after we started dating, Gavin admitted that he'd been afraid to tell me he was gay during that May visit, because if he'd guessed wrong about me, it would have ruined his residency.

The son of a doctor and the sixth of seven children, Gavin was a handsome twenty-six-year-old with thinning blond hair, green eyes, and a Martha Raye–like mouth, which he could purse into an adorable pucker or contort in comical ways. He looked great in photos, and had he been taller than five feet four inches he could have been a model. Although angelic in appearance, he had a vicious wit that could miniaturize the most imposing figure. He made me laugh when I should have been appalled; and he alarmed me when he raged to me about someone who angered him. He cursed like a sailor, drank like a fish, and smoked cigarettes, none of which I discovered until well into our courtship. In the early days he didn't exercise and had a bit of a belly. "We don't hike," he once said as I tried to cajole him into trekking to Kilauea Crater on the Big Island of Hawaii. In so many ways he was my opposite, but our relationship worked.

When he was on his eight-week internal medicine rotation, I manipulated the schedule so that we were occasionally on call at the same time. On the wards we behaved as colleagues, except for the long stare or wink across the ward when no one was looking. In the call room we were affectionate but never had sex. That would have been risky.

Our apartment in Old Town was on a tree-lined cul-de-sac, a mile east of my office and two miles south of St. Joe's. Most of the buildings were three- or four-story brick structures with imaginative facades artfully refashioned in the 1950s. The building we lived in had an arching entrance, bay windows, stained glass, friezes, niches with statues, and zigzagging passageways. Once a series of artists' studios, it was an oddly harmonious melding of art deco elements with those of a medieval Tuscan village. In front, a hodgepodge of inlaid granite and ceramic tiles—not a cement sidewalk—buckled from the serpentine roots growing underneath. It was a magical place on a magical street in an otherwise drab neighborhood. On this night, however, my apartment seemed more like a prison than an oasis.

As I came in, Gavin was already preparing dinner, and I could hear the clinking of utensils and pots. The nooklike kitchen had a serviceable oven, ancient refrigerator, cracked porcelain sink, and crooked, rotting cabinets, the only features that tainted the charm of the apartment. Although I felt nervous and my heart raced with anxiety, I hugged and kissed Gavin without any visible trace of distress. But I didn't bother with the usual end-of-the-day banter. Instead I blurted it out: Art had AIDS.

Gavin extricated himself from my embrace. "Who is this Arthur Sims, and why has he entered my life?" he said, glaring at me as if I were a dangerous stranger.

He paced the apartment, barking short responses to my questions and comments, tossing aside my attempts to console him, which made me feel alone and ashamed, for I needed consolation too. He was so distraught that I feared he'd pack his bags. I apologized repeatedly and struggled to soften the blow, but when you think you've accidentally poisoned the person you love, apologies are useless.

We eventually picked at our dinner in silence, the sharp sounds of cutlery and dishes on the tile piercing the air like shards of glass penetrating skin. My stomach churned like an acid-spewing caldron. When I looked up from my plate, Gavin turned away, staring at nothing and frowning. I gathered the dishes, glasses, and utensils and cleaned up the kitchen. We passed a sleepless night on opposite sides of the bed; even sedatives proved worthless. I would have swallowed the whole bottle to erase the horrors of that day, but I wasn't suicidal.

I remembered my first AIDS scare in November 1983, when I had a fever to 104, bone-breaking aches, and teeth-chattering chills that lasted two days. My white blood cell count was very low, like that of someone with an immune deficiency disorder. But then I broke out with a rash that covered me from head to toe—chicken pox! Or the time when I had pains in my fingers, wrists, shoulders, knees, and hips that I attributed to the toxic fumes Art and I had sprayed to get rid of the cockroaches in his apartment. That turned out to be an unusual manifestation of hepatitis B—I never became jaundiced or had dark urine. The hepatitis virus and the antibodies my immune system generated against it combined into microscopic crystals in my joints—*serum sickness* was the medical term. I'd had pneumonia also, back in late May 1981 just before beginning my internship. On graduation day I was so ill that the ceremony was a haze. Although I believed wholeheartedly in the precepts of the Hippocratic Oath, I had no recollection of taking it. Thank God I didn't see the CDC's report about a new disease in five homosexual men in Los Angeles until I'd fully recovered. Although I bounced back from all those relatively benign problems, that didn't mean I wasn't a medical time bomb.

The next morning, dragging ourselves to shower and shave, Gavin and I barely spoke to each other. Of course Art was in a worse predicament than either of us. Later that morning, Tom told me that one of the medical residents had informed Art of his diagnosis without consulting us or any other attending physician.

"You have cryptosporidium," she said to Art. "But don't worry, you will be OK."

Art, horrified, knew that wasn't true.

We were indignant at her impertinence and insensitivity. "I don't think she has any idea what the presence of cryptosporidium means," Tom said. It was clear that she meant no harm. Later we would educate her about the nature of opportunistic infections and their relationship to AIDS. But it wasn't her place to present a diagnosis of such gravity to a patient—even though residents are often the people called on to make life-and-death decisions in the hospital, such as "running a code" during a cardiac arrest. While we attending physicians poke our heads into a room for a few minutes and then disappear into an office, usually off site, the interns and residents remain in the hospital all day and frequently all night, dealing with scores of patients with all sorts of problems. Most residents are self-confident—which they need to be to win the trust of patients—but they can also be arrogant, lacking humility and sensitivity because they've rarely confronted their own failings. If a case goes badly, it's not their responsibility but that of the primary care physician or surgeon. They behave like know-it-all teenagers. Not that many years earlier I'd been like that too.

My indignation at what had happened temporarily shoved aside other emotions, but I suffered the next night and more, tossing and turning, torn by fear, anger, and resignation. I couldn't embrace Gavin, because he wrestled with the same feelings. For several days, touching him would have been like touching a cactus. But the needles gradually dropped off, and we became affectionate again. He forgave me, acknowledging that I wasn't at fault. We were both gay, both at risk for HIV/AIDS, and neither of us had intended to harm the other.

A few mornings after Art's diagnosis, I mustered the courage to visit him again, not as a doctor but as a friend, worried about how he was coping with his diagnosis. I was surprised to see his boyfriend, Max, in a chair at the bedside, crying. I didn't expect anyone else to be in his room at that early hour. Attached to an IV dripping at a furious rate and with a commode positioned strategically nearby, Art was despondent, staring at the floor and ignoring my greeting. He hadn't really believed that he had "the Big One."

Max wanted to talk. I quietly beckoned him to follow me. I guided him down the hallway, beyond Art's earshot. It was a typical morning on the ward. Most of the interns and residents were at morning report, yet the ward bustled with activity. Maria, one of the custodians, mopped the floor while another dried and buffed it to spotlessness. She wore a mask and gloves as she carried a plastic bag full of garbage out of a patient's room. Two nurses slowly pushed carts down the hall, dispensing medications. Hairnetted kitchen workers extracted breakfast trays from a large metal cabinet, the food made less appetizing as its aromas blended with the faint stink of the ward. Several attending physicians like me were also making rounds. No one paid attention to Max and me as we stood in the hallway, almost within kissing distance.

"Is he going to die?" Max asked.

It took me a few moments to respond. I hadn't come to Art's

room as a doctor, because I wasn't Art's doctor. I was his ex-lover, still roiled by conflicting feelings. But Max's unexpected presence caught me off guard, and his question jarred me back into that professional role. I stiffened my stance and switched mentally to doctor mode to answer him in the most compassionate—and emotionally distant—way that I could.

"Well, I don't know anyone who has survived," I said, "but I would never say anything's impossible."

"How much longer does he have?"

"I don't know. No one can say."

"Isn't there some medicine you can give to make him better?"

"We can treat some of the problems, but we can't cure the basic problem. There's no known cure for the problem with his immune system."

He wiped tears from his eyes.

"He thinks the world of you, Ross," Max said with such genuine sincerity that I was deeply moved. It occurred to me that I was no longer jealous of him, and I felt a pang of remorse for having once resented him. He was a loving, kindhearted person. If he feared for his own life, he didn't show it; he was concerned only with Art's health.

"Take good care of him," he said. "Please let him be able to go home."

I assured him that we would try our best, and I promised to relay the request to Tom.

Two weeks later, on July 4, I was awakened from an early-afternoon nap by a call from the hospital. The nurse told me that Art had had several episodes of "V tach," a potentially fatal rhythm disturbance of the heart, but had responded to firm thumps on his chest and a medication that restored his heart rate to normal. He was also on a drug to sustain his blood pressure. Relieved that he was still alive, I was perplexed by the call.

"Why are you calling me?" I asked. "Hadn't Dr. K. seen the patient?"

"No," the nurse said. "Your answering service said that you were the one on call."

That was true. When we opened our practice a year earlier, Tom and I had decided to alternate being on call by week. From Monday to Friday we rounded on our individual hospitalized patients. After the office closed for the day or on weekends and holidays, the one of us on call managed all our patients, making rounds and fielding emergencies. It was an arrangement that we felt increased the sense of personalized service, to distinguish our practice from others.

While technically I was on call this day, Tom had agreed to always manage Art's medical care after he was hospitalized, removing me from a potentially awkward situation. But Tom had forgotten our agreement. And now he wasn't home. I hadn't bothered to go to the hospital that day because I had no hospitalized patients—this was still in the early days of the AIDS crisis in Chicago.

I quickly showered and shaved, muttering with annoyance, calling Tom names that I would never have dared say to his face. Because I didn't have a car and considered it a waste of money to take a taxi, I walked. Ordinarily I walked everywhere, even on the most frigid winter days, and usually enjoyed it. My path to the hospital led me down our magical street and through Lincoln Park, past the zoo, conservatory, lagoon, and other scenic landmarks. Today was hot and humid, though, and I arrived at St. Joe's thirty minutes later irritable and soaked in sweat—but that might have been anxiety as much as humidity. I didn't know what I'd find or how I'd react when I saw Art.

I headed to the doctor's locker room and rinsed off my face with cold water, but my cheeks and forehead were still flushed and my hair was wet and disheveled. Once I cooled down and composed myself, I donned my gray coat, checked my pockets for their instruments, and rode the elevator alone to the fifth-floor intensive care unit. As soon as I entered, the nurses pounced on me with questions about Art's code status. Was he or was he not a "no code"? Art had signed a living will, which indicated that he didn't want extraordinary life support measures in the event of a cardiac arrest, but now he'd apparently changed his mind. I waved them off with annoyance but then calmly told them that I needed time to assess the situation. Inside I was furious that this decision had fallen into my lap.

I sat down at the nurse's station and browsed through Art's chart, attempting to piece together the events of the preceding two weeks. In that interval, Tom and I had barely discussed Art's case. A few days after my last visit, Art had developed a fever and shortness of breath. Tom consulted Dr. R., our pulmonary specialist, who whisked Art to the operating room and probed his bronchial tubes to obtain tissue samples. Those revealed two infections, PCP and a fungus called histoplasmosis. Alone, each of these infections would have indicated AIDS. Now Art had three opportunistic infections, two of which were difficult to treat, the other untreatable. It was crystal clear to me at that moment: his death from one or all three of these organisms was inevitable.

A floor nurse indicated in her July 3 notes that she'd discovered Art blue, pulseless, and unresponsive and called a code. The code team of several residents arrived quickly and was able to revive him with a flood of IV fluids and the application of an oxygen mask to his nose and mouth. There was no need to intubate him and place him on a ventilator or give him cardiac stimulants. He was transferred to the ICU.

Some time later the nurse who'd ordered the code admitted to me with shame and embarrassment that she'd been too afraid to give Art mouth-to-mouth resuscitation. She only pressed on his chest until the arrival of the code team. I told her not to feel guilty. I'm not sure how I would have reacted in a similar situation, performing the most distasteful part of CPR on a patient who was terminally ill with a dangerous and potentially contagious disease.

"It's unfortunate you arrived so soon," I said. "Nature should have been allowed to take its course."

The nurse nodded in agreement. But it was a moot point. Even if Art had been discovered lifeless hours later, when successful resuscitation was no longer possible, it's likely that the code team, abandoning common sense but claiming to honor the patient's wishes, would have gone further and intubated him, shocked him, and plied him with medications to restart his heart until Tom or I ordered them to cease.

For the rest of the day and night, Art remained in a "wakeful coma," eyes roving senselessly, arms and legs flailing aimlessly, unable to be roused or follow simple instructions such as raising his left hand or wriggling his right toes. Unexpectedly, he awakened the next morning and appeared to be behaving normally, although the nurses remarked that his short-term memory seemed impaired.

I approached his room with trepidation. He was a living ghost, stirring up a miasma of conflicting memories. Even in my darkest hours when I hated him, I never wished him dead. Ignoring a nearby cart loaded with protective gowns, masks, and gloves, I pushed open the door. The protection was unnecessary because I wasn't going to perform any procedures that would have exposed me to his body fluids. Moreover, if he'd already infected me with the AIDS virus, such protection wouldn't have mattered.

Art was pleased to see me and waved. I raised a hand in response but felt a momentary shock at his appearance. In only two weeks he'd become skeletally thin. No one had bothered to shave him in the three weeks since his admission to the hospital, and his cheeks were covered in a heavy overgrowth of black hair flecked with gray. A large encrusted sore festered on the left side of his lips. His skin had a gray death tinge. But his eyes, the final glimmer of life in a body ready for the grave, were a clarion blue and warm.

Looking past the tangle of IV tubes, bags full of futile treatments, and electrical cords, I noted on the cardiac monitor Art's rapid heart rate but stable blood pressure. A ventilator squatted ominously by the side of the bed, prepared for a full arrest. Outside his window was a view of the park and lake in full summer splendor. When I turned to him and asked if he remembered the preceding day's events, he seemed bewildered. I explained that he'd stopped breathing but was successfully resuscitated. His eyes widened and his mouth dropped open, as if only now he grasped his mortality and the inevitability of his death.

"I almost died?" he asked weakly.

"Yes," I said, "but I wouldn't expect you to remember those things. It's normal to forget that."

I asked him if he knew what was wrong with him. Puzzled, he squinted as if trying to dredge up a distant memory. Then he nodded his head as if he'd found the memory, but I realized that he hadn't.

"You have AIDS," I reminded him as gently as possible.

His face grew long, and he recoiled with horror.

"I have AIDS?"

"Yes," I affirmed.

"What are my chances of surviving?" he asked after a short silence.

"You're unlikely to be cured," I said.

"How long do I have to live?"

"That's something that only God knows," I said. "We can only guess."

Tears streamed down his face and he began to tremble. I squirmed with discomfort. This wasn't a conversation I'd planned to have with him. When I left my apartment an hour before, I'd hoped that he was in a coma so that I could zip in and out of the ICU.

"I don't want to die," he said with a sudden burst of emotion.

"I don't want you to die either," I said, my teeth clenching, my heart twisting, and a suppressed sob constricting my throat.

The next question was awkward, but I needed an answer. "Do you remember drawing up a living will?"

"Living will?"

He had no idea why I was asking the question. He'd forgotten all about a living will. The lack of oxygen had erased certain bits of knowledge and memories from his brain.

"Do you want to be revived and placed on a ventilator if your heart stops beating or you stop breathing?"

"Yes," he replied with such vehemence that I made no effort to dissuade him.

As we spoke, I bent over and rested my elbows on the guardrail, holding his hand. His fingers were bony and cold, unlike the flesh I'd touched and held years earlier. The situation seemed unreal to me. I tried to repress the memories and pretend he was just another patient, but that wasn't possible. Then he reached out and patted me on the head. My hair bristled underneath his palm.

"You're such a good person and I'm such a bad person," he said. "I love you and have always loved you."

This confession caught me by surprise. I felt myself blush. I'd once longed to hear those words from him, especially on those lonely nights when a simple phone call would have calmed my nerves and wiped away my insecurity. How much suffering they would have prevented! He spoke them only now, in the last stretch of his life, when it was too late. If we'd still been lovers perhaps I would have burst into tears, but my immediate reaction was to wonder whether anyone had witnessed this scene.

Tom and Gavin were the only members of the hospital staff that knew about my relationship with Art. And beyond the other gay and lesbian staff, no one at St. Joe's knew about my relationship with Gavin. To be an effective physician, I believed, I needed to command respect, not serve as fodder for gossip. St. Joe's, no different from any institution, was like a small town where privacy barely exists and everyone knows everyone else's business. If you weren't careful you'd wind up on a metaphorical tabloid, the most intimate aspects of your life revealed to the world. A person with a thicker skin and more audacity might have told everyone to fuck off. I still cared.

Fortunately the nurses, residents, and other ICU personnel were too busy caring for other patients to eavesdrop on our conversation. When I realized that I'd preserved my privacy and dignity, I ceased blushing and my bristling scalp relaxed. I felt guilty for not being able to reciprocate Art's feelings. A poor actor, I couldn't even dissemble.

"I care for you," I said in a voice that sounded cold and flat.

"Please be my friend," he pleaded. "You'll always be my friend, won't you?"

"Yes, yes, of course," I said.

I extricated myself from his grasp and examined him briefly, retreating into my physician shell, a far more comfortable space at that moment.

"How much longer do I have?" he asked again. "Weeks, days, months?"

Again I evaded the question. I told him not to think about that now and to rest. I patted him on the shoulder and left. Max had appeared at the threshold. Before closing the door, I turned around and saw Art wave to him. His expression was cheerful again, the feelings of anguish having vanished. I wondered if he realized that he was not at home. I also wondered if the words he'd spoken to me had any meaning in the context of an impaired memory.

Had I behaved more clinically and not been so self-absorbed, I would have performed a mental status examination, which tests a person's orientation to time and place, his memory, his ability to concentrate, and his judgment. I could have assessed the degree of Art's cognitive impairment and proved that he did or didn't suffer from dementia. But such an interrogation seemed pointless. His answers didn't matter and wouldn't have altered the outcome.

I wrote a short note and told the nurses that I would clarify his code status. When Max emerged from the room I took him into an empty conference room. We sat side by side. I was the doctor, he the patient's beloved; yet I could easily have been in his situation, in the same hospital, in the same conference room, but with Tom as the doctor, because there was no other doctor who cared for AIDS patients at St. Joe's in 1985. A montage of awkward and painful images briefly passed through my mind—I could imagine the nurses and secretaries snickering behind my back, their eyes and mouths twitching with scorn. It seemed impossible to me to have expected sympathy or shared grief. With a firm blink, I squashed these thoughts.

"I think you realize that Art's situation is hopeless," I said.

"Yes, I know."

"He stopped breathing yesterday and was brought back to life, but he's not quite the same person. His intellect is unchanged, he seems like Art, but there's been a significant change in his memory.

As you can see, he's actually blissful and in no emotional pain. He forgets as soon as you've stopped talking to him."

Despondent, Max stared at his feet. I wanted to put a comforting arm around his shoulder but hesitated. I looked around the room instead. It smelled of cigarettes. On a nearby table beside the ashtray filled with butts were open charts and loose paper notes. Someone had forgotten to remove an x-ray from the view box on the wall, but the image was difficult to make out because the light had been turned off. Through the window of the door I watched people move about soundlessly, as if in a silent movie.

"I'm so sorry to bring this up, but one of the problems we're having is that Art's code status is unclear," I said. "The nurses and doctors need to know how far to go. Do we put him on a machine to help him breathe if he stops breathing, or restart his heart if it stops again, or do we let him go? Right now things are halfway and we can't deal with life and death halfway."

"I don't know what to do," Max said tearfully. "Maybe I'm being selfish, but I think we should let him die. But he told me today that he wants to live, that he wants everything done. What do you think we should do?"

"It's really not my place to make that decision, Max," I said. "Unfortunately, it's up to you as his power of attorney."

He shook his head with indecision and started to cry. "I don't know, I don't know," he said.

"Maybe it's best if we make him full code," I finally said. "Art changed his mind and we should respect his wishes. If he weren't conscious, it might be different. But he's awake and still full of life. We'll do everything in our power to keep him alive."

"OK," he said.

"Why don't you stay here until you're ready to see him again. I need to speak to the nurses," I said as I squeezed one of his hands.

The charge nurse and the nurse taking care of Art that day anxiously asked me what to do if Art arrested. They were standing behind a curved desk that resembled the helm of a ship, from which all the rooms in the unit could be surveyed. A secretary listened closely to our conversation, reserving judgment at least until I was no longer present. I had a direct view of the door out of the ICU and desperately wanted to make a dash for it. Instead I told them that Art was a full code. If his blood pressure fell to dangerously low levels, give him medication to raise it to safe levels; if he stopped breathing, intubate him and put him on a ventilator; and if his heart stopped, shock him and give him whatever it took to get it going again. These were Art's new wishes, and Max wasn't prepared to go against them. If we didn't do everything we could potentially be sued, I said, even though Art would eventually die no matter what we did. The nurses reluctantly agreed that this was the best course.

As I was about to exit the ICU, I noticed a girl with blond hair standing alone at the back of the unit. At first I didn't recognize her, but then I realized that she was Art's oldest daughter, Karen. More than two years had passed since I'd last seen her. Now fourteen years old, she was blossoming into an attractive young woman. Waving tentatively, she gazed at me in helplessness. I had no idea how much she knew about her father's illness, and just the thought of explaining it to her in a manner that an adolescent could understand exhausted me. I gave her a hug, not from familiarity but in consolation. She told me that her sister and mother were parking the car and would arrive any minute. I made excuses to leave. I didn't want to confront Art's ex-wife.

Although I'd never met Alice, I'd caught glimpses of her through the windshield when Art and I would drive to the suburbs on weekends to pick up his daughters. As we motored up Alice would barely look at me, her pain evident from her avoidance of eye contact. It had been awkward for me too. I didn't end their marriage, but at that time I was her successor, a realization I deflected by looking the other way as if I were a mere passenger, not a lover. And now, as Art's life was ending, all sorts of uncomfortable and unwelcome feelings had returned. I was in no secure emotional state to deal with them.

I had no idea what Alice thought of me, or even if she would recognize me, and I didn't want to find out now. Oddly, as an ex I was in the same position as she, but that was something neither of us might have been able to acknowledge or discuss. I felt sorry for

Art's daughters, who soon wouldn't have a father. Whatever Art's deficiencies as a friend, husband, or lover, he was a conscientious, loving parent who never missed a child support payment and remained devoted to Karen and Molly long after his divorce. I left them behind with relief.

: 5 :

The Period at the
End of the Sentence
(1985)

Despite the unique personal and professional challenges Art's illness posed for me, Gavin and I didn't cancel our July Fourth party at our apartment. There were eight of us, including Tom. All but one of the guests were doctors. They arrived one by one. Ron, an internist at Cook County Hospital, arrived first, followed by Stan, who'd given up medicine to open a flower shop; Alex, an investment banker Gavin and I'd met on a trip to Key West; Ed, a dermatologist; and Bob, a third-year family medicine resident at St. Joe's, like Gavin. Bob fawned over Ed's leather boots and made everyone laugh when he dropped down on all fours onto the cold ceramic floor of the foyer and pretended to lick them. Leather drove him mad with desire, he proclaimed with sincerity.

We retreated to the overstuffed couches in the living room, talking over one another and laughing. From that vantage point we had a view of the surrounding units in the apartment complex, whose weathered brickwork reminded me of the architecture of San Gimignano, an enchanting, well-preserved medieval hill town a short bus ride from Florence.

Taking Tom aside, I whispered what had happened at the hospital. Expressing remorse, he said that he'd totally forgotten our agreement about Art. I wasn't sure I believed him. At first I said nothing to the others and tried to forget the traumatic events. Gavin served drinks and appetizers, and all was merry until the phone rang.

Everyone stopped talking. I faced a bookshelf, speaking softly into the receiver as if to the books, my back to our guests. It was a nurse from the ICU who informed me that Art had died. At that moment my mind went blank. I thanked her, asked no more questions, and hung up. Although I wasn't surprised, I hadn't expected his death to come so soon.

From my expression Tom guessed the meaning of the call, which forced me to talk about my experiences. My brief synopsis of Art's illness elicited murmurs of sadness from the group, especially when I let them know that he'd once been my lover. Gavin and I embraced, more from relief that the ordeal was over than from sorrow.

A few minutes later the phone rang again. The nurse apologized: Art was still alive! The doctors conducting the code had successfully resuscitated him, she said. Several of the guests gasped, and a pall descended on the festivities. We managed to carry on, but it was hard to enjoy ourselves. For the rest of the evening we were all Art, obsessed about our health. Such obsessions weren't unfounded. Within a decade, three of the seven of us would die of AIDS. The eighth, Alex, was so perturbed that we never heard from him again.

After our guests left, I received another call from the ICU. Art had coded again, and after twenty minutes the residents were unable to generate a heartbeat. Looking to me for guidance, they waited for a signal to stop.

"Enough's enough," I said. "Let him go."

I had no further contact with Max or with Art's family, didn't attend the funeral or memorial service in a distant suburb, and had no idea where he was buried. Had Art not reentered my life through his illness, I would have barely given him much thought. From an emotional standpoint I'd buried him long ago. Now I worried about what unwanted legacy he may have bequeathed to me, and what I might have bequeathed to Gavin.

I spent the next several months in various states of anxiety. Had I been infected, or had I managed somehow to avoid HIV? Art's death and its ramifications were too painful to confront head on. During the day, when hospital rounds and office visits distracted me, I could forget; at night I was haunted by the specter of my mortality. I constantly checked myself for signs of a deteriorating immune system—I looked into my throat for thrush, inspected my skin for the purplish lumps or bruises of KS. Sometimes I had night sweats, but that was a sign of stress, not disease, because I never had a fever, felt ill, or lost weight.

In the fall Gavin and I went to New York to see Larry Kramer's incendiary play *The Normal Heart*, a diatribe against a world that had failed to grasp the urgency of the AIDS epidemic before it spiraled out of control. As we sat waiting for the drama to begin, we scanned the whitewashed walls on which the names of the dead were emblazoned, a list that lengthened each day as the death toll skyrocketed. I didn't want my name up there. I didn't want to die of AIDS.

When the theater blackened at the end, it was impossible not to share Kramer's rage, which I directed at Art, at President Reagan, who'd barely uttered a word about AIDS, and at myself. Kramer called people to action, blaming all of us for making "a million excuses" not to get involved. I wasn't a firebrand; I couldn't be an activist marching in the streets, smashing windows, overturning cars, or brandishing placards. I was a doctor, and if I survived that would be my mission, my contribution to the cause: to be an AIDS doctor. I already was, but the epidemic in Chicago was in its early stages, not yet on par with New York and San Francisco, and I'd seen only a few dozen cases. I still viewed myself as a family doc, not a true specialist.

Before I could throw myself wholeheartedly into the fray, I had to know if I carried the AIDS virus. Unable to order an HTLV-III/LAV antibody test through the laboratory with which we contracted because the test was not yet commercially available, I contacted the Red Cross in early October to see if I could send samples from my office for screening. The medical director agreed. The first sample I sent was from a patient who, like me, wanted to know if he'd been exposed to the virus and had no signs or symptoms of infection. I was the second person tested.

The medical director told me that it could take up to two weeks to get a result. That seemed like an agonizingly long time to wait. Each day I checked the mail for a letter from the Red Cross and felt dejected each time I heard nothing. After a week I was almost paralyzed with fear. Imagining the worst, I assumed that it took longer to report a positive test than a negative one, because a positive result had to be confirmed with a more complex screen called a Western Blot. In anticipation, numerous scenarios passed through my mind: the reaction of Gavin, my parents, and the people I worked with at St. Joe's—all melodramatic fantasies and none based on fact. It was as if I had made myself Saint Sebastian, the martyr tied to a tree and riddled with arrows, or a religious outcast stoned to death for his transgressions. It was I who shot the arrows or cast the stones, not my imaginary assailants.

When the letter finally came ten days later, I let it sit on my desk for several minutes before tearing it open. My hands trembled as I extracted the two pages, the first with my patient's results and the second with mine. I broke into a cold sweat, and my moist fingers stuck to the envelope. They were ordinary pieces of paper, as if typed by a secretary. They hardly looked like the results I received from our laboratory, printed out by computer on striped pages and torn from a printer. It was hard to focus at first because I wasn't used to the format.

My patient's test was positive. Mine was . . . negative. For a moment I forgot about my patient as an immense wave of relief passed over me, ending months of anguish. Had I tested positive, I would have been shattered. It would have been a life- and career-altering event. I don't know if I would have found the strength to continue caring for my patients, especially my AIDS patients, knowing that we shared a common destiny, like inmates in a concentration camp watching their comrades perish in the gas chambers or hostages being hauled off one by one by their hooded captors. Not only had I been spared, but Gavin had also been spared. Had I been a man of faith, I would have thanked God for my good fortune. Instead I felt incredibly lucky. I showed the results to Tom, who hugged me with elation.

And then I realized that I had to confront my patient with terrible news. I wasn't in the frame of mind to deal with that nightmare at that moment, but I couldn't delay for long because I knew he was as anxious as I. Once I settled down, I called him.

From my earliest days as a physician, I've thought it best to be gently blunt when delivering bad news. Bad news is bad news, whether given in person or on the telephone, with no rules about how best to deliver it. If there's voicemail (or answering machine, in the 1980s) I refuse to leave ambiguous, potentially alarming messages ("this is Dr. Slotten; please call me when you have a chance"). Either I hang up and try again later or I report the results truthfully. After the revelation I offer to see the patient as soon as possible, ideally that same day so that we can talk frankly about a treatment plan—in the early days of the AIDS crisis, there often wasn't one—the prognosis, and the likely course of the disease. The conversation is at times a vain attempt to impose a structure on a process that doesn't have one and can quickly spin out of control. Despite thousands of such conversations over the decades, I've never ceased to dread delivering news that will forever change a person's life. Before picking up the telephone or entering the examination room, I've already imagined a scenario about the conversation based on what I think I know about the patient's character.

In this case, I didn't record my patient's reaction in my journal, and I don't remember anything about what must have been an excruciating conversation. I have a vague image of a tall, attractive man of about thirty sitting quietly in the examination room as I groped for words that treaded the fine line between hope and despair. Perhaps I held his hand after giving him the news, as I do now. He must have taken the news in stride, since he made no lasting impression on me. I couldn't predict his future. In 1985 we still didn't know that HIV was an automatic death sentence.

For some reason I looked at the results of the two tests again a few days later, just as one might check a lottery ticket to confirm that he'd indeed won the jackpot. To my horror, I noticed that my patient and I had been assigned the same confidential code. The birth dates and other demographic information on the forms were correct, but that sliver of doubt sent me into a panic. The director of the Red Cross couldn't completely satisfy me that there hadn't been a mix-up. I sent off a second sample, but since Gavin and I were about to take a three-week trip to Australia, New Zealand, and Tahiti, I would have to wait until I returned to the States to get the result. I told myself that the error was clerical and nothing to worry about.

In Australia we stayed a couple of nights in St. Kilda, the Boys' Town of Melbourne, a lively although rundown residential area on the beach, before heading by car to Sydney. Along the way we saw fairy penguins, koalas, and the occasional kangaroo and passed through Bible-thumping towns that reminded me of parts of the American South that I'd glimpsed on a whirlwind road trip when interviewing for medical schools in the fall of 1976. In Sydney we cruised around the scenic harbor; poked our heads inside the famous opera house, though it was the off-season; sunned ourselves on Bondi Beach; and spent two evenings on Oxford Street strolling in and out of gay bars, where the clientele differed little in dress and hairstyle from their counterparts in the US. We sat in a corner sipping beers as we listened to the same thumping disco music as in Chicago, not mingling with the crowd but enjoying the view.

From Sydney we flew to the South Island of New Zealand, once again renting a car and driving on the wrong side of the road from one picturesque town to another. In one the proprietor of our small hotel guided us to our room and said, in a vaguely threatening tone, "Two beds, which are essential, of course." Some antigay stories in the newspaper didn't reassure us that New Zealand was a tolerant country.

Our final stop was Bora Bora. Our hotel sat on the lower flank of the two-thousand-foot craggy, double-pronged peak that dominates the island. At night, under a bright moon, the mountain looked eerie, like Dracula threatening to envelop you in his raised robed arms. During the day it looked less menacing but no less formidable with its tangle of trees and vines and patches of bare rock. Along the flat road that rimmed the island we rode bikes one afternoon, passing little shacks with roofs of corrugated metal, pandanus palm leaves, or wood; clothes and trash strewn in the gnarled tropical greenery; and women who could have modeled for Gauguin, a flower tucked behind an ear and colorful tunics wrapped around their bodies. Remote and exotic, Bora Bora almost made me forget my anxieties.

When I returned to Chicago, the first thing I wanted to know was the result of my second AIDS test. I arrived at the office early, before anyone else, and waded through a pile of charts and papers on my desk, mostly laboratory and pathology reports, or notes about what happened to various patients during my absence. Buried somewhere among all this was my test result, which confirmed that I was definitely negative. That confirmation closed a chapter in my life; and the cord that tethered me to Art had now been severed. I could now move forward unencumbered in my role as an AIDS doctor.

: 6 :

Known Knowns

(1985)

Ⅰn August 1985, just one month after Art's death, Rock Hudson finally admitted that he had AIDS. For months there had been rumors about his declining health, which he and his publicists denied. Gavin and I watched him in an episode of the television series *Dynasty* and commented on his "AIDS look"—the hollow cheeks, sunken eyes, and wasted frame. The passionate love scenes with his costar Linda Evans created a sensation in the press, with accusations that he endangered the lives of Evans and other cast members. That was before it was established that kissing doesn't transmit the AIDS virus.

Hudson was the first major celebrity to announce that he had AIDS. Although he claimed that he'd acquired the infection through a blood transfusion, his homosexuality was an open secret. His death in early October raised awareness of the disease and doubled federal funding, though it was still far below what was needed to combat an epidemic. But the stigma of AIDS persisted, and AIDS forced many gay men out of the closet.

Not long after Hudson's confession, one of my patients, Gordon, a fifty-year-old professor at a state university, pressed a hand to his forehead in despair when it became clear that he had AIDS. Slumping in a chair in my exam room, he frowned with disgust as if smelling something foul or passing moral judgment on a murderer and exclaimed, "How ignoble! Why AIDS and not cancer?" That could have seemed pretentious, but Gordon was an erudite, dignified, and proud man, the opposite of ignoble. From his perspective, getting cancer was a matter of bad luck, but everyone knew how you get AIDS.

That word *ignoble* stuck with me. It perfectly captured how many of us felt about ourselves as gay men, how the world defined us, not by our accomplishments but by what we did in bed, which was considered dishonorable, base, shameful, and contemptible. Gordon was a perfect example. Most unbearable to him was the humiliating thought of revealing the secret life he'd led for decades to his evangelical Christian family in Kansas. For years he had lived quietly in a small university town in northern Illinois, where only his friend Louise, also a professor at the university, knew his true identity as a gay man. Now he feared that was all anyone would know about him.

Gordon had become my patient on the recommendation of Louise's mother, a nurse in the psychiatric unit at St. Joe's. A short, dowdy woman in her early sixties, she still wore a white uniform, white platform shoes, and the classic white nurse's cap over a hairstyle that hadn't changed since the 1940s. Arcs of black eyeliner replaced her eyebrows, makeup brightened her aging cheeks, and red lipstick clearly outlined the twin peaks of her upper lip. She was almost a caricature, a squat Nurse Ratchet from *One Flew over the Cuckoo's Nest*. Yet she was a motherly, tolerant, and caring soul who loved her daughter and wanted to help her daughter's best friend.

As Gordon's health deteriorated, Louise assumed more responsibility for caring for him. But the drive from the university, more than two hours from my office, was soon impractical once he could no longer get in and out of a car unassisted. And hospice care, which was still a nascent movement in the 1980s, didn't exist in their town. Louise cried when she admitted to me that she was overwhelmed. Without a larger circle of friends who could relieve her, he had no other choice but to return to his birthplace. It was a dreadful day when he closed down his apartment and headed back to Kansas.

But Gordon's elderly parents defied our expectations. If they had any faith-based prejudices against homosexuality, they cast them aside and cared for their son in their home until he died. Their dedication and devotion flew in the face of reports of AIDS patients being forced into homelessness by families who rejected them. From newspapers and magazines you could get the impression that the majority of families washed their hands of their AIDS-infected gay sons.

While most gay men with AIDS weren't homeless, now and then Tom and I did struggle to find a shelter for a patient, but not necessarily because his family refused to taken him in. Often these men needed twenty-four-hour care. Bedbound, they lost control of their bowels and bladder and developed bedsores or muscle contractures, which bent them into stiff pretzels; or, in the throes of dementia, they became combative and violent. Such care was more than some families, lovers, and friends could handle. What amazed me most wasn't the frequency of rejection and abandonment—it was the relative rarity.

For the first few years I didn't tell my parents about my work with Gordon or other AIDS patients. Not only did they not know about my relationship with Art, they knew nothing about the horrendous day I spent with him just before he died. My silence was about more than simply shame about being gay. I had long kept them in the dark about nearly every aspect of my life.

For the most part I'd had a happy childhood. My situation at home soured in adolescence, and not just because I was the typical sulking teenager, worried primarily about the pimples on my forehead. Our middle-class life had begun to crumble. My father and uncle had owned a small neighborhood store in Old Town called Economy Grocery. But in the 1960s, as supermarkets with endless aisles of food, copious bins of produce, and rock-bottom prices, threatened to drive friendly family-run stores out of business, economical it wasn't. Seeing the proverbial writing on the wall, they closed their city store and bought one in a northern suburb, where there was less competition. I helped out every Saturday, sweeping the sidewalk, stocking shelves, arranging an alluring display of apples in the front window, and using magic markers to create colorful advertising signs. Although promising at first, the move turned out to be disastrous. The previous owner had manipulated the books and swindled his sister investors, which an accountant had failed to catch until it was too late. Vendors hadn't been paid; taxes were owed; and my father and uncle were saddled with the debt to the sisters. My mother had become the store bookkeeper and was soon poking fingers into endless holes in a vain attempt to prevent the enterprise from imploding. They never caught up. Were it not for emergency loans from my grandfather and mother's brother, my father would have had to file for bankruptcy and give up our house, I learned years later.

My father, ordinarily mild-mannered and polite, turned irritable and snapped at me at the slightest provocation. I never seemed to be able to do anything right, which made me resent him and my ruined Saturdays. After a decade of struggle, the store failed. All the stress took a toll on my parents' relationship. Its effects on me were subtler. I developed an insecurity centered on money that persists to this day, which I believe is less about money than about the uncertainty of life itself. And my career—caring for men my age who were dying—had exacerbated that sense of instability and vulnerability.

In my teenage years my parents fought constantly and bitterly. Tables were overturned, plates and glasses crashed to the floor, and my father stormed out of the house, almost always over something minor. At one point I decided to assume the role of a mediator, but, as if trying to tear two dogs apart during a fight, I was chased away. After a while the fights happened so often we ignored them, although we spoke in hushed tones so as not to inflame my mother further. My father always returned after driving around the neighborhood for hours. The grinding sound of the garage door opening beneath my bedroom never failed to wake me up. After the fiftieth time, it was no longer reassuring; it was sad.

To calm her nerves, my mother started drinking two martinis every night, on the recommendation of her doctor. It was either alcohol or Valium. This was the heyday of tranquilizers, when the pharmaceutical industry touted medications like Miltown, Librium, and Valium as wonder drugs that offered chemical panaceas for what the feminist Betty Friedan referred to in *The Feminist Mystique* as "the problem that has no name," or the malaise of housewives. My mother, who never trusted doctors or their prescriptions and suffered not from uxorial malaise but the threat of homelessness, chose what she thought was the lesser of two evils. I wish she'd taken the Valium—at least she would have slept. In the evenings she often retreated to our home library, a martini glass in one hand as she thumbed through a magazine with the other. The shelves of the library contained a good number of Modern Library literary classics, which I cataloged after the Dewey decimal fashion, and an artfully displayed complete set of the *World Book Encyclopedia*. Most of the time it was my father's hangout, where he paid bills and swore at the TV when the Chicago Bears fumbled a football or the Cubs suffered yet another humiliating defeat.

I'm not sure what drew my mother to that room so regularly, but after two martinis it became a lair. When my brothers and I dashed down the stairs after finishing our homework to play pool or ping-pong in the basement, she'd stop me midstride, beckon me into the room, and urge me to answer a question, usually centered on whether or not I loved her. She didn't believe me when I affirmed that I did, perhaps because my answer seemed insincere to her. And maybe it *was* insincere, because I didn't like my parents much in those difficult years. We were not an openly affectionate family, even in better days. "I love you" wasn't a phrase any of us ever said to each other. I don't recall if she also stopped my three younger brothers to ask them a similar question, although I imagine she did. The drinks made her argumentative—and children never win arguments with mothers, even sober ones. As I endured her drunken accusations about my lack of respect for her ("You'd sell me down the river if you could," was one of her favorite jabs), every nerve in my body twitched violently.

My father, who had started drinking too, confided in me one afternoon while we were cleaning out the garage that he wanted a divorce. It could have been the perfect moment to bond and have a mature conversation about a momentous topic. Instead I looked down at the broom, probed for trash, and pretended not to hear him. They didn't divorce.

For refuge during these tumultuous years before my father's business collapsed, I fled to the house of my friend Doug. I spent almost all my free time with Doug, listening to records, experimenting with a chemistry set, or riding bicycles. My mother disliked Doug, an only child who had a learning disability, and felt I spent too much time coaching him through his homework. (Doug was highly motivated and eventually became an emergency room physician.) She also wasn't fond of Doug's parents, although they were always nice to me and treated me as a second son. Doug helped me through a difficult time in my life, boosting my self-confidence by lending an ear when I complained about how trapped I felt at home and giving the best advice a teenager could offer. Where I was timid, he was bold. He'd climb the tall elm tree in his yard and hang upside down from a branch, much to his mother's consternation (I can still see her clasping her hands at her bosom in distress), while I waited at the base, chicken that I was, ready to break his fall.

Doug spoke frankly about sex, which embarrassed me. When he told me that his father explained to him how to use a condom, I was taken aback. I couldn't fathom asking my father about that, or my father asking me if I wanted to know. He also told his mother about the petting he and I engaged in once in his bedroom one afternoon. Although she accepted such adolescent explorations as normal, she thought it best we stop. And we did. At first I was embarrassed. Then I was ashamed and angry at what felt like a betrayal. I'd never been in the habit of sharing my deepest emotional thoughts and experiences with either parent. I didn't feel a need for an intimate relationship with them, and my parents didn't seem to know how to have an intimate relationship with me.

Luckily, I felt, I'd gotten into college in California, as far away as I could arrange to go. I spent five years there—flying back to Chicago was too expensive to do more than once a year—further distancing me from my parents. During my freshman year a few of my dorm-mates cried because they missed their families, but I stared at the ceiling without emotion, wondering if there was something wrong with me because I didn't feel sad. I dug deeply into myself, searching for something to make me cry. I couldn't find it. Two thousand miles from Chicago, the membrane that had begun to envelop me in adolescence as a response to turmoil at home hardened into a carapace. That sense of isolation, reinforced by complete financial independence from my parents—scholarships, loans, and a twenty-hour-a-week job in the food service covered tuition, room, board, and other expenses—had nothing to do with being gay because I didn't know that I was.

Returning to Chicago for medical school in 1977 brought me no closer to my parents. Getting to their home by public transportation involved a twenty-minute hike to the L and another forty-five minutes to travel to the end of the line. From there I could walk another hour or wait to be picked up. Once I was there, we talked about the weather, food, politics, national news, and the doings of my brothers, cousins, aunts, and uncles, but when it came to my personal life I was more evasive and uninformative than ever. By this time I did have something to hide, my sexuality. That subject never came up in conversation.

Eight years later, not much had changed. Until one September afternoon in 1985. It was cool and cloudy, and the three of us sat in their dimly lit dining room with its white shag carpeting, wood-paneled walls, and tasteful contemporary and midcentury modern furnishings. By this time my parents had turned their lives around, the grocery store dumped at a loss and their loans repaid. They'd both obtained real estate licenses and now made enough money to go out for the occasional dinner and even travel abroad.

My father, a handsome sixty-year-old with a head of hair a thirty-year-old would have envied, relaxed on a wicker sofa in one corner, his left foot curled under his right knee. In another corner I stretched out on the black-leather armchair with my feet on the matching ottoman, slowly swiveling from side to side. My mother rested her elbows on the teak dining table, reading a magazine. She was an attractive woman in her late fifties, petite with chestnut brown hair and a minimum of makeup. Closing the magazine, she looked at me over the rim of her reading glasses. A beaded chain hung from the glasses' arms like the outline of jowls, which made her look like a prosecuting attorney about to cross-examine a witness. It was an expression that often put me on edge, triggering the metaphorical walls to rise in a flash and protect me.

"Your brother J. has good taste in women," she said, for no obvious reason. "But they only look at him as a friend."

Thoughtlessly, I made an unflattering remark about his appearance that related to some of his persistent eccentricities, which I thought explained why women weren't attracted to him. I immediately felt small and petty, but it was too late to retract. My mother's eyes narrowed and her lips flattened, the top one pressing down onto the other as she rose to his defense. My apology did nothing to mollify her. A decade earlier my brother had plunged into a major depression after discovering his college roommate in the throes of a mental breakdown. He took a leave of absence for six months to undergo psychotherapy before returning to complete his studies. I'd steered the conversation into dangerous territory, like a soldier in war who's forgotten that he's driving over a minefield.

In a bold and quizzical voice my father suddenly asked, "Do you think you'll ever get married?"

The question caught me off guard. I broke out in nervous laughter. Blushing angrily, I looked at both my parents for a brief moment before turning away. My mother was still scowling, and my father raised his eyebrows in genuine curiosity. I felt like a warthog on the African plain, stalked by lions—defiant but vulnerable, possibly standing his ground but prepared to flee. Thoughts flitted through my brain: *Should I tell them ... no ... well, yes, here's my chance ... I dare not ... they know more than I think ...*

"I suppose someday," I lied, convincing not even myself. "But there's so much else I have to do. I don't have time to date. I'm too busy building a practice."

My mother wasn't going to let me get off that easily. "Are *any* of your friends married?" she asked.

She listed all of my acquaintances she knew who appeared to be single. I thought of one physician friend my parents and I had run into during a neighborhood garden walk. He had a swaggering gait and spoke in a harsh Chicago accent. He stood with legs spread and arms folded—the picture of a macho man. It would have killed him if he thought strangers could tell he was gay. "Is he *married*?" my mother had asked later, not fooled for a minute.

I swiveled in the chair to avoid her gaze, a hint of sweat moistening my forehead and my heart racing.

"What about Doug?" she asked. "Will he ever get married?"

Once more I was caught off guard and laughed. Among my friends and acquaintances he was one of the few straight ones, although his somewhat effeminate gestures—he had spidery arms and legs and walked, as a friend once observed, as if pulled forward by a string attached to his belly button—and the fact that I'd spent so much time with him in high school made my mother think otherwise. If she'd named anyone else, I would have confessed.

"I would think so," I said, thinking of the many sexual conquests he bragged about. "He's something of a Casanova."

"You two have a *special* relationship," she said, lowering her glasses to the tip of her nose.

"We do not!" I protested. "He's my best high school friend and that's it."

"How often do you see him?" she challenged.

Before I could answer, she launched into a tirade about his rude behavior when Tom and I celebrated the opening of our practice a year earlier. At the reception he ignored my mother, whom he disliked as much as she disliked him, and he left without saying goodbye. It wasn't our supposed secret relationship that irked her but his insolence.

"This is leading nowhere," my father interrupted. "Let's change the subject."

My father, who'd launched the perilous conversation, saved me in the end. Grateful, I retreated back into my shell. But without saying as much, we had settled for don't-ask-don't-tell. They knew that I was gay; I knew they knew; and they knew that I knew they knew. That was the last time we discussed my marriage prospects.

But this uncomfortable confrontation had nothing to do with

marriage. It was an awkward attempt to break through my shell, and I evaded my parents ineptly. Two of my brothers were already married. Whether that deflected my parents' concern about me I don't know, because we never talked about it. J. never would marry. As time passed, Gavin was gradually absorbed into my family, and his large family gradually absorbed me. That absorption occurred without drama, at least in our presence. We entertained everyone at Thanksgiving; he was invited to a seder at Passover—the only Jewish holiday we celebrated, albeit a bit irreverently since half the guests weren't Jewish; I spent Christmas with one of his two sisters and their children. As time passed we were accepted on both sides as a couple, even if nobody discussed what we were—don't-ask-don't-tell wasn't just a Slotten thing. That unwritten policy applied to many gay men and women of my generation.

And no one in our families ever brought up that other taboo subject—AIDS.

: 7 :

The Saga of Stan S.

(1986–88)

I met Stan at a small dinner at Tom's apartment in November 1983. I don't remember the conversation because I was too self-conscious about my face, which bore the fading effects of chickenpox. My condition embarrassed me even though Stan was a former dermatologist. But we were at a party, and I was gay and vain.

A few years earlier, in his mid-thirties, Stan had quit his medical practice to devote himself full time to his floral business. When I was in medical school, I lived close to his shop in Old Town. I'd pass him on the street, but as he set out the bins of flowers and plants, he ignored me. Evidently I wasn't his type. An attractive man in his early forties, he had a wiry, muscular frame with bowed legs, large balding head, long thin nose that curved toward his mouth, which in profile made his face appear almost flat, neatly trimmed mustache, and introspective green eyes. He strode with purpose and conviction, reminding me of a cowboy who'd just dismounted his horse. Glassy eyed with admiration and jealousy, we young gay doctors marveled that he no longer needed to practice medicine. In an era when many physicians had catapulted into the economic ranks of the top 1%, that was quite an achievement. We weren't jealous of his wealth; we were jealous of his life. He made just as much money pursuing his dream, which was less stressful than being a doctor. We were less courageous.

During the next two years Gavin and I spent an increasing amount of time eating out with Stan in the neighborhood. Our banter ranged from medicine to politics, his latest boyfriend and, of course, AIDS. By 1985 he'd left his first store after a dispute with his business partner and opened up a new one on the Gold Coast, not far from where Art had lived. Stan didn't think of himself as a florist but as an entrepreneur who sold flowers. A florist, he said mockingly, is a fussbudget with lisping speech and a mincing gait whom people ridiculed behind his back. He took great pains to buck that stereotype. I laughed at the image because I knew what he meant. I viewed myself as a physician who happened to be gay, not as a gay physician. In a climate of bigotry, it was an important distinction for me to make. At the time I believed that my profession and identity were mutually exclusive, the former taking precedence over the latter.

Like any great businessperson, Stan had a keen eye for what sells. He made sure that the quality of his product and lavishness of display outclassed those of all those fussy florists he dissed. It worked. The political and social elite of Chicago flocked to his store. And if they demanded, as they often did, discounts and special services, he was not intimidated. As far as he was concerned, A.L. and E.K. could (I paraphrase him here more politely) shop somewhere else if they wanted a discount—but there was no better place for flowers. Each month the dollars piled up like an ever more fruitful harvest; much of the cash he stashed away in cabinets and cubbyholes in his apartment, out of sight of nosy tax collectors. When he showed me his secret hoard, I was shocked by his brazenness. I would never have cheated the IRS, even if I grumbled about taxes—but that's why I'm a doctor and not a businessman.

Stan was also a perfectionist, a trait I admired. Like a scientist or economist, he kept a daily calendar recording temperature, weather conditions, and money collected, and he compared year to year, month to month, and week to week, acquiring a feel for the market. A wilted flower or ragged display raised his ire so as to send his employees scurrying for cover. But he was generous and kind, paying his staff good wages and treating them as if they were members of his family, and they were fiercely loyal to him. Moreover, he pitched in, ringing up customers, putting together bouquets like an artist working from a palette, and hauling plants off delivery trucks with the ease of a stevedore.

Stan once invited me to Kennicott's, a market where he bought most of his flowers. He liked to go early, before other vendors had picked over the newly delivered stock from across the country and Europe. We drove to a grimy, industrial part of Chicago I'd never seen before. No doubt my father had come to a similar neighborhood to select his grocery's produce and procure the freshest meats. Stan rejected anything less than perfect—and purveyors at Kennicott's, in fear and out of great respect, kowtowed to him—which impressed me because so many flowers at other stores seemed flawed: a brown petal, a torn leaf, or buds that never bloomed. Taking only seconds to examine each specimen, he tossed aside flowers that I would have bought without a thought and pointed out their imperfections like a botanist. I had no idea how complicated it was to make a flower shop first rate. The experience affected my attitude toward my own practice. I too longed to be the best at what I did.

Stan cultivated many friends and acquaintances within the city, nationally, and across the seas. Some were professional, such as his friendship with dermatologists at Northwestern, where he had trained. Some were business, as with the Kennicott brothers or art dealers he met at auction houses when he began to dabble in American Impressionist art, paying for paintings with wads of ten- and twenty-dollar bills exfiltrated from his apartment. Others were sexual. His sexual appetite was clearly voracious, and he had had hundreds of liaisons over the years. Occasionally he had relationships, but these had rarely lasted long. He guarded his privacy with even greater rigor than I did and had difficulty with intimacy and affection.

When Gavin and I befriended him in 1983, Stan had hooked up with Rob, a handsome man fresh out of college with sandy hair, sparkling green eyes, a dimple on his chin, a muscular build, and (most important to Stan) the demeanor of a frat boy whom few would have suspected of being gay, for Stan was still in the closet with everyone except his closest friends. By that time Stan was terrified of AIDS; casual sex with numerous partners had become too risky. His only reason for sticking with the relationship, he claimed, was fear, not love. Before Rob he'd never had a steady lover. After two years they were fighting, though whenever we got together at our apartment, eating and talking at the blocklike dining table with its artful checkerboard pattern, there wasn't the slightest hint of disaffection. They laughed, grabbed each other's hand, and bumped shoulders like any couple who adored each other. Gavin and I laughed, grabbed each other's hand, and bumped shoulders in loving sympathy.

But in reality they never really got along, and their parting in 1987 was bitter. Unfortunately they lived next door to each other, a circumstance that drove Stan crazy. A creak at Rob's door sent Stan to the peephole to spy. When he heard laughter and music through the walls, he suspected that Rob was trying to make him jealous. But why was Stan jealous, I wondered. Telling us that he had never enjoyed sleeping next to Rob after sex, he provided details about his dissatisfaction that were comical but made us blush. Cuddling bored him; awakening with a lover brought him no solace or comfort. Stan didn't have an ounce of romance, which had frustrated Rob. Although he filled his store with roses for Valentine's Day, Stan scoffed at presenting flowers to a lover for any occasion. Sex for him was like eating, a necessity of life. Once he cleared his plate, he was sated. In many ways Stan was more of a guy than a gay.

Stan's paranoia about AIDS grew slowly. In the spring of 1985, while we were guests at his tastefully decorated vacation home in Key West, he had an upper respiratory infection that became a chronic cough. He complained of being short of breath. I hadn't brought my stethoscope and couldn't listen to his chest, but it was evident that he was just congested. Already I'd seen a good number of young men who were short of breath, wasting away, and desperately ill. Stan, who appeared robust and kept pace with us as we attended afternoon tea dances, cruised the bars, and dined out without any difficulty, didn't resemble them. Eventually his shortness of breath resolved, but he feared that any ailment heralded AIDS. He was one of the unfortunate guests in my apartment the day Art died in July of that year. A more frightened group of men could not have been assembled on a more inauspicious day.

One by one, his past loves, friends, and acquaintances suc-cumbed to AIDS. Scott, who owned a B&B in Key West, died igno-miniously in a hospital, Stan said. Scott had developed dementia and incontinence, but his doctor never stopped testing and treating him, adding meaningless days to a tragically shortened life. When Stan visited Scott for the last time, Scott no longer recognized him, which crushed him. Stan wasn't one to cry, but there were tears of anger in his eyes when he described Scott strapped to a bed in an adult diaper. I didn't fault the doctor. To give up all hope in a young man seemed almost criminal in those early days of the epidemic. Sometimes we couldn't believe what we were seeing: a man with a bright future cut down like a soldier by a bullet, as if his life had no purpose. At least a soldier could conceivably die for some greater cause.

Another friend who died of AIDS was Christian, a Parisian. Stan had introduced us during a trip to Paris in June 1986. Handsome and loquacious, with a winning personality, Christian charmed us immediately. He dressed so well—shirts and pants that perfectly conformed to his slim body and stylish shoes—that we looked like country bumpkins in comparison. It was clear that he and Stan had once been more than friends.

Gavin and I had traveled to Paris that summer to attend the sec-ond International Conference on AIDS, though it was a convenient excuse for visiting the most beautiful city in the world. Stan, who shunned all medical conferences now that he was no longer a prac-ticing physician, didn't attend but caught up with Christian and other acquaintances he hadn't seen in a few years. The conference, which lasted three days and brought together twenty-eight hundred scientists and clinicians from all parts of the globe, generated few headlines because there wasn't much to report. The biggest news was the revelation that the major mode of transmission of HIV in Haiti was heterosexual, proving that everyone, not just gay men, was at risk. The greatest disappointment was the pessimism that an effective vaccine could be developed in the foreseeable future. HIV didn't behave like influenza, mumps, measles, smallpox, polio, or many other viruses that could be rendered harmless with antibodies; it defied neutralization. In April 1984 Margaret Heckler, the US secretary of health and human services, had announced the discovery of the cause of AIDS and raised hopes by predicting that there would be a vaccine against it within two years. She was wrong.

I was still thrilled to be at the conference. At family practice conventions I was the outsider, the lone gay family doc wandering upstream past schools of straight people, genuine family physicians, practitioners who treated traditional families: newborn babies, rambunctious kids, sulking teenagers, newlyweds, pregnant women, struggling parents, and doting or dotty grandparents. My families were unconventional: two men or two women trying to make a life together in a hostile heterosexual world; or two gay men, one or both dying of AIDS; or the single gay guy looking for love, trying to dodge the plague.

Now I was part of a larger community of like-minded people who were medical pioneers and shared a common mission, battling what would soon become one of the great epidemics of modern times. We weren't in the spotlight yet, and expectations were low. That would change the following year, when the conference was held in Washington, DC. At the opening session, protestors would symbolically turn their backs on Vice President George H. W. Bush, who represented the Reagan administration. With what appeared to be regal indifference, Ronald Reagan rarely mentioned AIDS in addresses to the general public—a silence that diminished its urgency and seriousness. From that point on, the International Conferences on AIDS became magnets for activists and reporters who broadcast their increasingly angry protests as the death toll skyrocketed and politicians either turned a blind eye or denied the global catastrophe altogether. Thrust into that maelstrom, I knew once again that I'd found my calling.

A year after our Paris trip, Stan came to the office for his annual checkup. Since he felt well and had no physical complaints, I expected to find nothing abnormal. But when I looked inside his mouth I was startled to see white patches, a sign of a seriously impaired immune system. I said nothing and continued, listening to his heart and lungs before pressing on his abdomen as I engaged him in casual conversation. Although I maintained as placid an expression as I could, my mind was in tumult. I must have masked my feelings well, because he sat unperturbed and asked no questions. But I was uncertain how to proceed.

The world of AIDS medicine had been changing. In March 1987 the FDA approved AZT for the treatment of people with the worst form of the disease. That approval generated near hysteria in the gay community and among their doctors. It was the first bit of good news on AIDS. Although not touted as a cure, AZT promised to add precious months or years to a person's life. Patients now flocked to my office for testing. But that's not why Stan was here. Despite his great fear of AIDS and his near certainty that he'd been infected, he refused to know his HIV status. The onus of bringing up the subject fell on me.

I could have been blunt: *Stan, you have thrush, which means you probably have AIDS, and I want to prescribe AZT, but I can't unless I know for sure that you're HIV positive.* But Stan wasn't the type of person who responded to orders, even from a well-meaning friend. And only on rare occasions was I blunt—for example, if a patient with appendicitis refused surgery or one having a heart attack refused hospitalization. But with less certain outcomes I settled for a softer approach. I nonchalantly offered to test him since I was ordering routine bloodwork anyway. If by some terrible chance he were positive, I said, we at least had AZT now.

"Absolutely not!" he said. "If I ever get AIDS, I'm jumping out the window. I could never live like that."

I was taken aback. If I tried to persuade him to take the test, I'd have to explain why. If I explained why, he might literally jump out a window. Choosing to avoid an unpleasant confrontation with uncertain consequences, I reluctantly let the matter drop. Somewhat to my relief, this difficult conversation would have to wait until another day.

A month later, at the end of August, Stan called me in a panic after noticing the yeast infection himself. I asked him to come to the office immediately. As he sat on the exam table like a nervous little boy, feet dangling without touching the footrest and hands rustling the paper with anxiety, I studied his throat carefully without showing signs of foreknowledge. When I withdrew the balsawood tongue depressor and placed the light source back on the wall, I hesitated. Despite having mulled over a thousand times what I'd say to him when the day of reckoning inevitably arrived, I was unprepared.

There's a good reason doctors are advised not to treat people they love: they can't be objective. But AIDS wasn't cancer or heart disease; it was a disease unique in history, for most of those who contracted it in the United States and Western Europe in the 1980s were gay men. In the West, AIDS and being gay were almost synonymous; cancer and heart disease were seen as having far less to do with one's identity. As a result, the majority of caretakers of their fallen friends were gay men or lesbians. Although I could have referred Stan to a handful of other colleagues who now dealt with AIDS patients, Stan and I were enmeshed. Referring him elsewhere would have been tantamount to abandonment just when he needed me most. I felt duty bound to stick by him, no matter how awkward or heart wrenching.

After I confirmed that he had thrush, our gazes locked and the terror in his eyes pierced me to the core. It was like standing on the shore as a man thrashed in the water and having no means to save him. This feeling of helplessness and impotence would cleave to me until the end of Stan's life. To throw up my hands in despair and admit that I felt helpless would have been useless to him. No one wants to hear that, no matter how true it is. I had to appear strong and steadfast while preparing myself psychologically for the worst.

Frantic, Stan agreed to allow me to draw blood to check the status of his immune system, but he continued to refuse an HIV test. I didn't argue with him because it didn't matter: A yeast infection in an otherwise healthy person could mean almost nothing other than that he was HIV positive, and he knew it. When the results came back a few days later, they confirmed that he had severe immune deficiency. When I gave him the news over the telephone, he didn't jump out a window. Much to my relief, he agreed to AZT.

Still, Stan focused on AZT's side effects instead of its benefits. An eternal pessimist, he was also a former doctor who'd seen horrible allergic reactions to, and even death from, medical treatments. The botched surgery, the missed or incorrect diagnosis, and dangerous drugs—when you've witnessed the worst, it's difficult to acknowledge how much good modern medicine has accomplished. No wonder doctors and nurses make terrible patients! I tried to convince Stan that the benefits outweighed the risks. In my opinion, AZT was better than doing nothing and watching him die. Even if its effects lasted only a few months, I said, AZT offered a tiny ray of hope. I spared him the logical end of that sentence—"in a hopeless situation."

Only days after starting Retrovir, the brand name of AZT, two tablets every four hours around the clock on a rigid schedule, Stan complained of headaches, fatigue, and nausea, among other physical complaints, and searched for any excuse to avoid taking the recommended dose. I pleaded with him to do everything in his power not to change the dosing. Never a radical in medicine, I've always followed the rules (or guidelines, to use more professional language) until or unless solid data dictate otherwise. Occasionally during the height of the AIDS crisis I lost a patient to another doctor because I was too "conservative," the patient would say, as if I were still leeching, when in fact experimental or nonconventional treatments scared me because they could be lethal.

At dinner one evening, Stan coughed incessantly, as if he had a bad cold or bronchitis. A few days later, when he called to tell me that he became short of breath climbing stairs in his store, I offered to drive him to the emergency department at St. Joe's. I now owned a car, which was less a reflection of my increasing income than an acknowledgment that walking to and from my apartment, the hospital, the office, and patients' homes with black bag and stethoscope in hand was inconvenient, time-consuming, and even absurd. The purchase was a major concession to a more complex life that Gavin embraced with a sigh of relief. A Mercedes Benz, the car Stan drove, was beyond our reach; I'd settled for a Toyota Corolla.

As we trudged from the garage to the ED, Stan stopped frequently because of fits of coughing and a feeling that he might pass out. Looping my right arm around his left to ease the strain and provide support, I inched with him toward the intake desk. By this time the emergency room nurses weren't surprised to see me with an AIDS patient—and he'd hardly be the last that I'd accompany there. We maneuvered him into a wheelchair and pushed him into a private room, where he changed into a gown, hoisted himself onto the uncomfortable gurney, and lay down, huffing and puffing from the effort. I asked the nurse to start an IV and hook him up to oxygen, and ordered some bloodwork and a chest x-ray.

Because he was in no mood for talking, I left Stan for a while and chatted with the nurses and lone physician. It wasn't a busy night. The secretary occupied himself with paperwork. A patient moaned behind one of the closed curtains; from behind another I heard the bleeping of a heart monitor. A technician rolled a cumbersome x-ray machine into Stan's room and then left a few moments later. I wrote a note in the ED chart about Stan's condition.

Fifteen minutes later the tech notified me that the film was developed. I crossed the hall to the viewing room and positioned the flexible celluloid rectangle the size of a placemat onto the viewing screen. It showed what I feared: fluffy white patches scattered throughout the black background of his lungs, a pattern most consistent with PCP. When I showed Stan the chest x-ray at his request, holding the image up to the fluorescent ceiling light and pointing out the infiltrates, I told him that he needed to be admitted.

"What choice do I have?" he asked.

I promised to do my best to make him better.

Stan wanted me to get his robe, toothbrush, and slippers from his apartment. While a private room was being arranged for him, I drove back through Lincoln Park to his high-rise a mile south, wondering how this would turn out. If he had PCP, he was likely to improve after intensive treatment. By 1987 we'd gotten better at preventing early death from this disease. But PCP was tricky because it sometimes killed despite everything we did. I hoped that he might have a bacterial pneumonia, which would be easier to treat. In either case, no matter what he had, he was entering a death spiral.

I was concerned that Rob would hear me fumbling with the keys, open his door, and ask me questions Stan wouldn't have wanted me to answer. Fortunately, he wasn't home. Walking through Stan's apartment in his absence, I felt as if I were a trespasser in a museum after hours, my footsteps echoing off the freshly waxed parquet floors. Stan had created an elegant living space, with antique furniture intermixed with more contemporary pieces. His walls were full of original high-quality artworks. Before entering his bedroom, I noted the Picasso lithograph on the wall next to the door.

Stan had painted the bedroom walls evergreen, which made it dark and cozy. In a corner he displayed a magnificent cactus on a pedestal, its stems budding like prickly mycelia in every direction. On the dresser next to his bed was a photograph of his parents on their wedding day. Near the closets hung a painting of a Black Madonna, the only religious symbol in his apartment, chosen for its beauty and artistry rather than for its religious significance. Long ago he'd given up Catholicism. He professed no allegiance to any religion, and his illness didn't drive him back to God. He had nowhere to turn for spiritual solace. And on that level I could be of no help.

Opening the closet doors in the bedroom of Stan's condo, I was shocked by the disarray. Stan had piled one thing on top of another. The slovenliness seemed uncharacteristic because he was fastidious in every other way. A cockroach scurried out of sight. I didn't have the heart to tell him later. Grabbing a robe, I shut the doors before something else might jump out, and returned to the hospital. But he told me I'd brought the wrong robe. The one he wanted hung on the back of the door in the bathroom.

The next few days were difficult. The samples from the bronchoscopy—performed by Dr. R. with sedating doses of Valium and Demerol, which were barely adequate to reduce the anxiety and discomfort of a tube jammed down the throat into the bronchial trees of the lungs—confirmed PCP. Dr. R. was a hero to me. Since the beginning of the epidemic, he had never expressed any fear about his personal risk of HIV infection, which was real—he was exposed to infectious body fluids during every procedure—or "moral" objection to the patients he treated. He had an extraordinary work ethic and seemed never to sleep. He might appear at a patient's bedside at 10:00 p.m. on a Friday, or whisk a patient off to a bronchoscopy at 3:00 a.m., after an arduous day that had begun early the previous morning. Without him it would have been impossible for me to make an accurate diagnosis of and treat lung infections related to HIV. I am forever grateful to him. Treating people with HIV requires collaborating with other healthcare providers, and I relied on Dr. R. more than on almost any other consultant at the time because pulmonary complications from HIV infection were very common.

Stan complained about his severe sore throat after the procedure and whispered, wincing at every word as if swallowing shards of glass. We'd already agreed that the family practice or internal medicine residents wouldn't follow his case, which meant that I was called for every problem, day and night. I loved him dearly and would have done anything for him, but he was one of several hospitalized patients I had. I had a packed schedule at the office, telephone messages to answer, and paperwork as well. There was only so much time I could devote to him without feeling exhausted and overwhelmed.

The hospital care angered him. He chased nurses out of the room and writhed when poked with a needle for a blood draw or insertion of an intravenous line. A nurse who took his pulse with her fingers pressed on a gauze pad to guard against transmission of HIV—a ridiculous gesture because checking the pulse posed no risk—humiliated him and infuriated me. To his chagrin, a customer of his store recognized him when he was walking the halls, although most of the time he stayed in his room as if it were a bunker. The medication prescribed to treat his pneumonia upset his stomach, but he couldn't tolerate antinausea medications. In short, it was a miserable experience for everyone involved.

Once discharged to his apartment, Stan said that he felt worse and begged to stop his medications. I told him that he needed to be treated for a total of three weeks, as long as the side effects weren't worse than the PCP itself. Unable to sleep, he called me multiple times a day to rage about the world. After completing his therapy, he felt better and his chest x-ray had cleared up. This news lifted his spirits a little. But his fevers soon returned, as did a staccato cough.

One night Gavin and I visited him when he wasn't feeling well again. As we sat in the kitchen table making small talk, Stan suddenly pressed his palms to his temples, stood up, stamped his feet like a toddler throwing a temper tantrum, cried out, and ran to his bedroom. It was shocking to behold, a display of raw, uncensored emotion that I'd never seen in Stan before. It was useless trying to console him. He refused to talk, and we didn't dare enter his room against his wishes. We heard muffled sobs through a wooden barrier that was just one inch thick but separated us by a chasm. His anguish was heartbreaking, the more so because it was beyond consolation. Embarrassed, he ordered us to leave. We had no idea what else to do, so we did. But I couldn't shake the sight and sound of that unexpected outburst. I knew it would be seared into my brain for as long as I had a memory.

As we exited, all sorts of images of how I'd behave in a similar situation flashed before me. I was afraid to die too. Art had frequently confessed to me that he thought the worst way to die was to be stabbed with a sharp knife. That was long before he knew that he had AIDS, a death worse than a stabbing, in my opinion. People sometimes say that they're not afraid of death itself but dying, with its attendant suffering. They hope to pass away in their sleep, presumably without any conscious knowledge that they're about to die. But I'm afraid of both—the suffering and the finality. (One of my college professors, an old-fashioned field biologist, said that he wouldn't mind dying if he could poke his head up from the ground every ten years to see what was happening in the world. I liked that idea, to glimpse how the world changed in ten years, a hundred years, and even a thousand years.) Witnessing other people's deaths in the prime of their lives made me no less fearful. To maintain a facade of courage or equanimity in the face of one's own imminent demise, as in the movies, requires a degree of inner strength, or superior acting skills, that I lack.

The next day, calmer, Stan agreed to hospitalization to evaluate the fevers and cough, but he refused another bronchoscopy and wanted to be treated as if we knew the diagnosis. Unfortunately, his white blood cell count had dropped to a dangerously low level, putting him at risk for life-threatening infections that had nothing to do with AIDS. With such a low count, he couldn't go home and had to remain in isolation in a hospital room. Although we didn't have to wear masks, we gowned and gloved if we needed to touch him—to protect him from us, not the other way around—and disposed of these items in a special container when we left the room. He was also forbidden from eating fresh fruit, which couldn't be sterilized. Eventually he accepted the bronchoscopy, which proved negative for PCP and other causes of pneumonia. After further testing, we concluded that he had had a reaction to the treatment of his PCP, which was reassuring because he'd recover.

The next two months were more peaceful. Stan regained his strength and sense of well-being. He became more hopeful and tried to be optimistic, even cheerful. Remarkably generous, he sent us huge, magnificent plants as housewarming gifts (we'd just moved from the apartment on Burton Place to a townhouse we purchased west of Boys' Town). Each plant must have cost a lot, even with his industry discount. When we visited his store one day, he insisted that we take numerous handwoven decorative baskets. His generosity bordered on mania. We sat in his cramped office—its walls lined with shelves full of vases, his desk piled with bills and papers, a print of Van Gogh's irises adorning the wall above, a pastel drawing of his shop by an aspiring artist that rested on a wooden bench behind his swivel chair—laughing, joking, and discussing politics. His laughter was truly joyous. He'd throw back his head, mouth wide open, showing his white teeth, his eyes observing you for a reaction. It wasn't a belly laugh—Stan could never relinquish total control—but a good-natured, warmhearted laugh.

This period didn't last long. Soon he noted gradual loss of vision in his right eye. I referred him to my ophthalmologist friend Dave, who discovered that CMV was the cause of his encroaching blindness. Stan complained of the unfairness of it all, comparing himself to Christian, who seemed to have no problems with his HIV infection after recovering from PCP. Tom and I had managed to procure Christian several months of AZT, which we shipped to Paris because AZT was not yet approved in France. But Christian's invincibility was an illusion, because he was destined to die like everyone else with full-blown AIDS. Stan showed me an article from a French newspaper about an experimental HIV treatment; after this he hung all of his hopes on this therapy and made dozens of calls to Christian, with whom he pleaded to get him into that program. But the diagnosis of CMV disqualified him.

A new medication had recently been approved to treat CMV, but it interacted with AZT. Administered through a vein, it would have to be given multiple times daily indefinitely, and Stan could no longer take AZT. Stan's only other option was to be referred to a specialist at a university who was engaged in a study that involved giving the medication in the eye. Because only a small amount of the medication would be absorbed into the bloodstream, he could stay on AZT. Stan didn't want to go blind, didn't want to die, and didn't want to stop AZT. But it really wasn't much of a choice. He might not lose his eyesight, but he would die no matter which procedure he agreed to.

The local injection involved shoving a needle through the eyeball to deliver the medication directly to the retina. It was a brutal procedure, despite the application of a topical anesthetic to the eye. Dr. P., the ophthalmologist, was a Nazi as far as Stan was concerned, callous and unsympathetic to his plight. Sitting for hours in the waiting room that he shared with a variety of patients, mainly elderly men and women with cataracts and glaucoma, he waited in dread until summoned. A medical assistant brought him back to an examination room, where he was placed on a table. Gowned and gloved, the doctor entered, described what he planned to do in a perfunctory manner, anesthetized the eye, injected the drug, and moved on to the next patient. The doctor's barbarity, as he described it, obsessed Stan.

Unfortunately Stan suffered a common complication of CMV, a retinal detachment. Dr. P. admitted him to the hospital for reattachment. To ensure success, Stan had to be put at complete bed rest, lying on his stomach for a day with a cumbersome patch over his eye. Terrible as that was for him, the crowning blow came when Dr. P. told him that CMV was now also in his left eye. The message was delivered without passion or compassion, Stan said. After giving the news, the doctor walked out of the room.

Stan was furious, feeling completely destroyed by the news. There was absolutely nothing I could do. I had no professional relationship with Dr. P.; I'd never met or spoken to him; and I was in no position to influence his behavior by threatening to refer patients elsewhere, because he offered a service that no one else in Chicago did at the time. Without treatment Stan would have gone blind. I appealed to Dave, but Dave was also HIV positive and couldn't afford to alienate Dr. P. Stan finally agreed to stop AZT and receive his CMV treatment intravenously.

It surprised me that Dr. P. had shown no sign of respect for a fellow physician. A little kindness, a friendly chat about Stan's education and training, why he'd given up medicine, and so forth, would have gone a long way in easing Stan's anxiety. I concluded that Dr. P. was at best insensitive, like a good number of other doctors I knew, interested only in accruing subjects for a clinical trial to enhance his reputation, puff his curriculum vitae for future governmental or pharmaceutical grants, or supplement his income, but indifferent to the patients in the study. Perhaps AIDS and gay men disgusted him; or if we grant him a bit more humanity, he erected a harsh facade because he had no idea how to behave around a mortally ill patient.

In the end it didn't matter. Stan's health rapidly deteriorated, and as he declined he became unexpectedly docile. The personality change was evident when he reported to me blandly that he thought he was having seizures. Several times he'd awakened on the floor or in bed in a pool of urine, his tongue roughly bitten, he said. Alarmed, Gavin and I rushed to his apartment and found him soiled and disheveled. After cleaning and dressing him, we drove him to the hospital. A scan of his brain showed a pattern consistent with PML, an untreatable viral infection. Soon he became confused and could no longer control his bowels and bladder. Then he lapsed into a coma, surrounded by the family he avoided and a few friends who loved him.

Stan had barely talked to me about his childhood and family, and what little he revealed was disparaging. Born in Chicago, some-where on the southwest side in a predominantly Polish neighbor-hood, he once said that he was proud of his background because he came from nothing and pulled himself up by the bootstraps to be-come successful; but he was also ashamed because his parents were ignorant, uneducated, and incapable of understanding him. When I met his mother and sisters—his father had died years earlier—they indeed seemed less sophisticated and not as well educated as he. Both sisters were overweight and dressed without any concern for style. His mother was a demurer, diminutive figure. Whereas Stan had cultivated a refined midwestern accent, they spoke with a Chicago twang. But there was a clear physical resemblance—the shape of the head, the curve of the nose, the wary laugh. And they were pleasant to deal with and grateful for my care and support of Stan. The diagnosis of AIDS didn't seem to faze them.

What happened in childhood to cause Stan to harbor such ill will toward his family remained a mystery to me. Growing up gay in an immigrant community in the 1950s, where neighbors, teach-ers, parish priests, and even your parents made it clear that homo-sexuality was a sin or worse, must have been unbearable to him. Moreover, he was bright and ambitious, with aspirations that may have clashed with his parents' expectations. Somehow he wound up at Colorado State, or "Ski University," as he called it—a strange choice for a lower-middle-class student, though not for one who dreamed of a more glamorous world. Whatever the reasons for his deep-seated animosity, I felt sorry for his family because Stan had excluded them from his life. He also excluded them from his will.

Stan had finally come to terms with the inevitability of his death from AIDS and revised his will during the brief period after the PCP but before the CMV. Desiring some sort of legacy, he asked my advice about what to do with his investments, which were substantial. His lawyer and I sat with him at his kitchen table one evening developing a plan. On the wall behind him was a colorful elongated painting by a Haitian artist that portrayed a funeral procession, which was more festive than funereal. But it was hardly a festive moment. I wanted to grab his hands in sympathy, but he wasn't the touchy-feely sort. Once he made up his mind about something, he was all business. He left no room for sentiment.

Knowing that Stan was adamant about not leaving anything to his mother or sisters, I suggested that we try to fill a gap in the care of those infected with HIV by creating a unit somewhere for the terminally ill who had nowhere else to go in the final stages of their illness. Stan liked the idea and left me in charge of a sizable amount of money to make it a reality. Working with Horizon Hospice, one of the first hospice organizations in the United States, I initially hoped to establish a freestanding facility. But because of the high cost and uncertainty of such a venture, the board and I decided instead to find space at Chicago House, which housed homeless HIV-positive people, at the time mainly gay men. The unit was named after Stan, and for several years it provided compassionate end-of-life care in a homelike environment.

The last twenty-four hours of Stan's life were agonizing. His family, Gavin, our dermatologist friend Ed, and I were all present for the deathwatch, sitting around the bed in the private room I'd arranged for him. Each time he appeared to stop breathing, we let out a collective gasp of relief. But then he'd breathe again. This type of breathing appears painful but it's not, because by that time all higher cognitive functions have shut down; only the basic functions of life persist. Yet it is still awful to watch, even for me. Time expands into an eternity. As the clock crept toward midnight and then beyond, Stan's breathing became shallower and less labored. Toward the end, his mouth opened and closed but almost no air entered or exited his body; this is known as the "O sign." He finally died in the middle of the night, his tongue protruding slightly from the side of his motionless mouth—the "Q sign"—as our eyes burned with tears and exhaustion.

Pointlessly I went through the motions of examining him. I checked for a pulse, made sure his pupils didn't react to light, and listened with my stethoscope for the faintest of heartbeats. I had to look like I was doing something important, but it was an illusion, a secular substitute for a sacred ritual once performed by a priest or other religious figure. Stan lay lifeless, glazed eyes staring vacantly into space, skin still moist from sweat, lips drawn apart, and teeth coated in dried saliva and other matter. I rearranged the covers, drawing them over his ashen arms and chest.

We all stood near the bed in stunned silence for a few minutes. I expressed condolences to Stan's mother and sisters, my words sticking in my throat, and then hugged each of them. Ed looked at the floor and shook his head, clicking his tongue against the roof of his mouth in distress and disbelief. Gavin wiped tears on the back of a sleeve.

I didn't cry—I usually don't in such circumstances. It's not that I didn't feel sad; I felt terribly sad that Stan—my friend, my patient, and my mentor—was dead. But crying isn't my go-to emotion when crying is the expected response, especially in public. It makes me feel like a cold person, but I'm not. I can cry. I cry during an emotionally charged movie or while reading a good novel with characters an author has magically made me care about—but only when I'm enshrouded in darkness or alone, unwitnessed. In the final moments of *La Boheme*, Rudolfo's piercing note of despair at the realization that Mimi has died never fails to bring me to tears, no matter how many times I swear that I won't get choked up. The clashing, atonal crush of horns—an orchestral evocation of a final exhalation—gives way to a haunting melody in a minor key as the tenor sobs out the name of his beloved. Those notes and her name burrow into my unconscious and dredge up what otherwise I can't seem to summon to the surface at the appropriate moments in the real world.

Stan's death was senseless, wrong, and unfair, just like all deaths at a premature age, whatever the cause. If I learned anything from that experience, it was that when you faced the reality of your own imminent death, you could go down kicking, screaming, and raging at the world or as stoically and quietly as Sydney Carton on his way to the guillotine in *A Tale of Two Cities*. It doesn't matter. The end is the same.

: 8 :

The Predator
and Prey Within
(1991)

On Thanksgiving morning 1991 Gavin and I, flanked by armed scouts, trudged through the African bush with four others, all very hung over from too much wine. The moans of an unseen lion jarred us to attention and made us forget our pounding eyes and heads. For a moment I wondered who was the weakest of us in our group, the most likely to be attacked after the guards scrambled up a tree to save themselves. Crowding together, we tiptoed on the path, snapping the dried grass and slapping the muddy earth with our boots, a dead giveaway to the beast in the bush. But the lion didn't give a shit about us, and we soon became aware of our bodies again, sweating in the searing heat, having foolishly forgotten to bring water. A fetid hippo pool dotted with menacing periscope eyes beckoned us. No one dared, of course.

In the evening Jeannie, a stout, jovial elderly British émigré who with her husband managed a camp on our ten-day tour of Botswana, prepared a kind of Thanksgiving feast for us. With no turkeys available, she roasted a duck and cooked a pie of squash and sugar. How odd and wonderful it was to celebrate Thanksgiving. I had so much to be thankful for—most importantly, just being alive. Only a week earlier I'd been in Chicago grappling with conflicting emotions of relief and remorse as I waited to board the plane. I was like a soldier longing for his furlough while feeling guilty for abandoning his comrades in the midst of a war. And it was a war by this time, against an enemy as invisible and implacable as that lurking lion. My comrades weren't other doctors but my patients. For them this Thanksgiving wasn't a day of thanks for life but one more waystation on an inexorable march toward their death.

———

On the morning of my departure for Africa, I had bolted out of bed at 6:00 a.m. as usual and rounded one last time on my patients on the AIDS unit. I could have taken the entire day off, but I felt dutybound. Their plights haunted me. I couldn't shake them from my thoughts, no matter how excited I was about traveling to the Okavango Delta. Although I had full confidence in Tom and our new associate C., I felt responsible for my patients.

By 1991, 11 West at St. Joe's had been in operation for three years. As the AIDS crisis escalated, our wards began to overflow with the sick and dying. Before 11 West, no HIV-positive patient at St. Joe's was allowed to share a room with an HIV-negative one, although you can't catch the typical infections afflicting a person with AIDS by sharing a room, except tuberculosis. (Non-AIDS patients often posed the greater health risk to AIDS patients' suppressed immune systems.) You also can't catch AIDS from a toilet seat or touching faucets and sinks. In that era, while you wouldn't have heard a peep from patients if they shared a room with a serial killer, if they shared a room with an AIDS patient it would have been a public relations disaster for the hospital.

In the earliest days of the epidemic, the hospital staff feared people with AIDS as much as the general public did and fabricated any excuse not to treat them. One surgeon I worked with sent a patient with an inflamed pancreas to x-ray every day to get a picture of his abdomen because he was afraid to touch this patient's body. A gastroenterologist begged me not to refer any more AIDS patients to him for a colonoscopy because he had two young children to raise and didn't want to put himself at risk of infection. A thoracic surgeon, the chief of surgery at St. Joe's, left me in a quandary one night when he refused to operate on a patient who suffered from purulent pericarditis, where pus fills and constricts the lining around the heart like a vise. If the pressure was not relieved, my patient would die. "Ask one of the younger guys," the surgeon said before abruptly hanging up. With an anxious eye on the heart monitor, I ripped through the hospital directory in a frantic search for a surgeon who wouldn't blow me off. I found one and to this day I remain indebted to him.

Ordinarily I don't hold a grudge. But I couldn't forgive those other physicians for abandoning me and my patients in the hours of our greatest need. For years I avoided them at staff meetings, refused to greet them in the hallway or doctors' lounge, and never referred a patient to them again.

Because of so much antipathy toward AIDS patients, it made sense to create a safe haven for them. HIV-infected people required a dedicated and compassionate team of healthcare providers— doctors, nurses, nurse's aides, and social workers—to manage a complex array of medical and psychosocial problems. In their final days, weeks, or months, they needed compassion, not rejection. St. Joe's wasn't the only hospital in the city with an AIDS unit, but we followed closely on the heels of Cook County and Illinois Masonic Hospitals.

Setting up the unit had taken months of hard work, including overcoming prejudice against gay men at St. Joe's, which, paradoxically, because of its proximity to Boys' Town, seemed to have a larger-than-usual number of gay and lesbian staff members— administrators, nurses, file clerks, technicians, doctors, and priests. In 1988 Tom and I lobbied the nuns to establish the unit, appealing to their commitment to the marginalized and underserved. After they agreed to the concept, we attended interminable round tables with administrators who, though well meaning, relished turning molehills into mountains. Each meeting ended without a decisive plan, pushing the opening date of the unit further into the future. Trained to make decisions based on experience, knowledge, and even instinct because a patient's life often hangs in the balance, doctors are an impatient bunch, and I was no exception. After each of these futile meetings I wanted to scream. In my opinion, we could have accomplished in one meeting what hadn't yet been accomplished in five.

While we waited, we courted patients and philanthropists from the gay community to donate money for renovating the rooms and creating a homey lounge with refrigerator, television, bookshelves, couches, and chairs. We set aside another room for hospice care, one large enough to accommodate lovers and families, who could spend the night comfortably on a convertible sofa bed or recliner. To our delight, we had no trouble raising money. Our patients and their families were remarkably generous. In gratitude, we made sure that plaques honoring them adorned the walls of 11 West.

In anticipation of final approval, we assembled a group of healthcare workers, mainly nurses, social workers, and nurses' aides who already worked in the hospital, whose sole job would be to care for AIDS patients. And then one day 11 West opened, not to any fanfare but suddenly, as if by the flip of a switch. The CEO, who was tired of hearing us complain about the delays, made it happen. Patients were moved, personnel shifted; and—voilà!—a wing of the hospital became the AIDS unit. It wasn't the wing we wanted—we preferred 11 North, with some rooms that had scenic views of Lake Michigan and Lincoln Park—but it would have been ridiculous to complain. We were grateful that we were given an entire wing, which could hold up to twenty patients at a time. When the remodeling was completed a few months later, 11 West, with its gleaming linoleum floors and tastefully decorated rooms, welcomed our AIDS patients with open arms. I felt proud. I was to spend the next fifteen years there, often heartbroken, occasionally inspired.

———

One of the patients I had rounded on before departing for Africa was David. Before this latest hospitalization I'd seen him so often in my office for various problems that he seemed more like a friend to me than a patient. He now called me Ross instead of Dr. Slotten, a sign of affection as well as respect. This would be the last time I'd see him alive. Pausing at the room's threshold in my gray coat, I scanned the clipboard on which his vital signs were recorded.

His blood pressure had dropped to dangerously low levels, and in compensation his heart beat at a very high rate. Nearly every organ was failing: his kidneys had shut down so he produced no urine; his heart pumped ineffectually, compounding his inability to shed fluid that accumulated in his lungs, belly, and legs; and his bone marrow had stopped producing blood cells, essential for carrying oxygen and fighting off infections.

With a sigh I entered David's room, which was silent except for his labored breathing and the hissing of oxygen. In response to my questions about pain and comfort, he grunted a few un-intelligible words that were muffled by the plastic oxygen mask pressed against his nose, cheeks, and mouth. I leaned over his bed in a fruitless effort to understand him. Staring at his wasted arms, torso, and sweaty body, I recalled when he was robust and vibrant and the prospect of dying seemed remote. Now the moment we had dreaded for months approached. Struggling under the mask to catch his breath, he'd turned an indescribable shade of gray, a color between the pink of life and the blue of death. I squeezed his hand with affection but didn't receive the usual response. Letting the limp, cool, and swollen fingers slip from my grasp, I stroked the stubble of his beard with the back of my hand. "Goodbye, David," I said softly and left the room.

There were so many others like David in my practice now, though none at the time so close to death. Those men would still be here when I returned from Africa, but they'd already begun their journey down a path whose tracks were vanishing like footprints in wave-washed sand. *Such sadness, such unbearable sadness*, I thought. I kept hearing Kurtz's words from Joseph Conrad's *The Heart of Darkness*: "The horror, the horror!" Although those words were uttered in a different context, they still resonated for me as I left David's bedside and the ward. The horror, the horror! I imagined my hands pressed against my skull like that Edvard Munch portrait of a woman screaming on a bridge. Like her, I wanted to run away from a living hell.

By 1991 I'd lost hundreds of patients from AIDS, and the number increased with each year. June 5 had marked the unofficial anniversary of the epidemic, ten years since the Centers for Disease Control published its report. Since then 180,000 AIDS cases had been reported in the United States; there were more than ten million cases worldwide. The statistics boggled my mind. AIDS was now the second leading cause of death in American men between the ages of twenty-five and forty-four, after accidents. It was the leading cause of death in my own practice.

By a coincidence I didn't consciously seek, I was heading to a continent ravaged by AIDS. Botswana was among the countries hardest hit by the epidemic, but I tried not to think about that. I wasn't going there to study the impact of AIDS, at least not this time. I followed an urge to explore the world while escaping my present. I hoped that the hiatus would reenergize me, because I felt enervated, exhausted by my work caring for the sick and dying.

Yet I was conflicted. How frivolous of me, I thought, to leave on a holiday, brimming with excitement, when these men had no hope of seeing the next year. It was the kind of guilt that sprang not from any religious conviction but from my mother, who would reprimand me as a child for wasting food when there were millions starving in India or as a senior in college for throwing away money on a grand tour of Europe when I could be investing in real estate instead. I was supposed to be a penitent, flagellating himself at every thought of pleasure.

Despite the Jewish guilt—a concept my mother didn't believe in—I could continue practicing medicine only if I interrupted my working life at strategic intervals when my spirit flagged. A cliché like "Life is short" became a mantra of survival. Delaying gratification until some imaginary retirement date seemed absurd to me, when so many men my age were dying decades before their time. I didn't want to look back on my life with regret, cursing myself for putting off the dreams I could have pursued in my prime. Although I was HIV-negative, I behaved like someone who walked through the valley of the shadow of death, not fearless but fearful that the end was near, that the moments of good health were precious and shouldn't be wasted.

In the weeks preceding our vacation, I buried myself in as much literature as I could find on Botswana. This was my fourth trip to Africa. Books about the continent lined my shelves like cairns marking my past visits — three times to the national parks of Kenya and Tanzania — or sentinels guiding me toward future destinations. Now I'd visit the south. All these books shared one thing for me: in darker moments, they were refuges insulating me from the barrage of demands, anxieties, frustrations and self-doubts that threatened to overwhelm me. Sometimes, in an obsessive fit, I'd pick up the *Lonely Planet Guide to Africa* and read the section on Botswana over and over again.

Books weren't my only emotional outlet. When distraught, I often went straight to the piano, an upright my parents had bought me when I was a child. After I returned to Chicago from California, this beloved instrument followed me from apartment to townhouse to single-family home as I moved around the city. Often I spent an hour or more lost in a world of beautiful sound, pounding the keys and running the arpeggios of a Chopin nocturne or Schubert impromptu as I vented feelings of despair about the cruel fate of my patients, my own mortality, or, in the case of my former lover Art, the abrupt end of a tumultuous relationship. At such moments I felt like a lab rat that pushed a lever repeatedly to get its fix of cocaine.

Although I could have gone anywhere in the world — a Mexican beach or an island in the Caribbean might have made more sense — Africa beckoned me once again. The lure had less to do with the pristine wildernesses and wildlife inhabiting them than with something more primal. Because humans evolved in Africa, Aaron Latham wrote in *The Frozen Leopard*, Africa was in our genes. Peter Matthiessen, in *The Tree Where Man Was Born*, put it more poetically: "Perhaps it is the consciousness that here in Africa, south of the Sahara, our kind was born."

In a different life I might have been an archaeologist or fossil hunter, unearthing our origins like the Leakeys. Each discovery of one of our ancestors piqued my interest and provoked speculation about our place on the planet and in the universe. Even an atheist like me, dealing with issues related to death and dying every day, contemplated such metaphysical questions.

How I became a doctor is still mystifying to me. Before college I'd had no firsthand experience of what it was like to be a doctor. No members of my immediate family were physicians. My father's father had sold cigarettes for a living during the Depression; my mother's father had been a tailor. No one except my father had finished college, and none were professionals. In high school I founded the Aesculapian Club (Aesculapius was the Greek god of medicine; his serpent-entwined staff remains a symbol of medicine today), partly at the instigation of Doug, who always wanted to be a doctor, and other friends in high school. A local orthopedic surgeon mentored us and rounded up colleagues to speak to us about their experiences. One of my heroes at the time was Dr. William Nolen, who wrote a best seller, *The Making of a Surgeon*. I had the opportunity to interview him at my high school during a book tour in Chicago. Otherwise, what I gleaned about medicine had been from television shows like *Dr. Kildare, Marcus Welby, M.D.* and *Medical Center*. These popular shows, with their handsome stars, idealized the role of the doctor in a secular age when science promised answers to all of life's questions. Through their brilliance and uncommon wisdom, those TV doctors saved lives and solved people's problems. Dressed in their surgical scrubs or long lab coats, they embodied the notion that medicine is a noble calling. I didn't want to own a grocery store like my father (nor did he expect me to). I wanted to save lives and solve people's problems like Dr. Nolen and my television heroes. I had no idea that I'd chosen to pursue one of the most difficult professions imaginable. Saving lives and solving medical problems would be infinitely more complex than anything I ever dreamed of at the age of seventeen.

––––––

From Chicago we flew to London and then to Johannesburg. Our route took us over the great sights of Africa: The Sahara Desert, the Nile, Mt. Kilimanjaro, the Rift Valley, the Congo River and Victoria Falls — all shrouded in darkness or hidden under heavy cloud cover. What other continent boasted so many iconic landmarks, I wondered. I became nostalgic about previous African trips and fantasized about future ones. There were so many possibilities. If only we could take a break from life and get this wanderlust out of our systems! *Two years would be enough, just two years*, I pleaded with my superego, which wasn't amused. *No!* chided the stern inner voice with the intonation of my mother, and out poured a litany of rationalizations that included ridiculous words like *responsibility* and *money*. I retreated timidly to another plane of thought.

From Johannesburg we flew to Botswana and boarded a four-seated bush plane piloted by an ebullient white man named Charlie who looked too young to fly. "Buckle up," Charlie reminded us, but when I told him that my seatbelt was broken, he shrugged and said, "Oh well, that's Africa, you know." Charlie guided the plane effortlessly, as if driving a car over invisible roads and unfazed by the atmospheric equivalents of potholes and surface irregularities. I watched for the lone raptor that might inadvertently collide with us, mucking up the propeller in a whir of blood and feathers, stalling us and hurtling us to our deaths. But the sky was empty except for clouds that unrolled swiftly above us.

"Elephant!" Charlie suddenly cried. "Do you see them?"

He tilted the plane sharply to give us a view. Gavin slid toward me, and I gripped my seat with fingers curled into talons. Several gray lobules with flaps splashed through water, lumbering silently along. *OK, OK*, I thought, *just fly the damned plane*, but I feigned excitement and praised his game-sighting skills. After twenty minutes the landing strip came into view, a swath of green amid brush and woodlands. We circled sharply and descended. After landing, my entire body vibrated and my blocked ears felt like the inside of a seashell.

Our first camp was rustic, like a frontier outpost. An older white man, plump and smiling, welcomed us. His spindly legs poked through khaki shorts, and he wore a khaki shirt with epauletlike straps. His hair was short and wavy, and his complexion was ruddy. He seemed like someone who could wield wit as quickly as a fearsome temper. Clive made an amiable quip about our being "bloody Americans." His wife Barbara, with dirty fingernails, extended a hand for us to shake. She too was in her mid-fifties. Big-boned, tall, and no longer slender, she had an attractive square face and lively green eyes accentuated by crows' feet. Her skin, a toasty brown, was leathery from too much sun.

Clive and Barbara, who'd fled Zimbabwe after the end of British colonial rule, weren't fans of the government of Botswana, or any African government for that matter, although Botswana was the only true and stable democracy on the continent. Products of the imperial past, they dismissed Africans as incapable of self-governance. Their aim was to stir up enthusiasm for wildlife preservation, though they were pessimistic about Botswana's future.

We walked with them through the compound and strolled along the edge of the plains. The camp, an oasis of safety and comfort, was on our left; on our right, Africa, where only the fittest survived. The sun at its zenith, hot and blinding, pressed down on us, obliterating our shadows. An antelope foraged, but most animals had retreated into the shade. This was Africa, touched only lightly by humankind.

"Too many people in Africa, I'm afraid," Barbara said unexpectedly while gazing at the limitless horizon, shading her brow. "But now there's AIDS. Perhaps that will save Africa. It might be a godsend."

I froze in my steps, knees locked and teeth clenched, as I looked at the landscape but saw only terrible images in my brain, skeletal bodies prostrate on mats or bare earth in some remote African village. AIDS doesn't resemble starvation, where imploring eyes beg for food; AIDS eyes are too sick to implore.

Whose Africa was AIDS saving, I wondered: that of the white colonialists who'd been turned into nomads or that of the Africans themselves? The continent had been invaded, colonized, and divvied up into artificial countries, creating the chaotic conditions from which AIDS emerged and thrived. That was too fraught an issue to discuss with people I hardly knew and at whose mercy I'd be for the next few days, but perhaps this was merely a way to start a conversation. It must have been obvious to them that Gavin and I were partners. How silly of us to pretend otherwise—or maybe not. Such is the treacherous life of the gay traveler, guessing at motives, seeing shadows that don't exist, or missing messages that truly intend harm.

"AIDS is a problem in the West," I finally managed to say. "But it's even more devastating in the third world, where dissemination of information is next to impossible and where behavior will only be changed after it's too late."

"Condoms don't work around here," she asserted. "The men absolutely refuse to wear them. And the women are powerless to say no. I've heard that nearly half the Zimbabwean army is infected with the AIDS virus."

Barbara was right about the high infection rate and the reasons for AIDS's explosive spread throughout the continent. At a future international conference on AIDS I would hear one scientist proclaim that Robert Mugabe's failure to address the public health catastrophe in Zimbabwe should be treated as genocide or a war crime. Forget the fact that he ruined his country economically, the scientist said; Mugabe would be remembered as a leader who turned his back on his people and let hundreds of thousands of them die of AIDS.

As we returned to the large communal tent, I could have launched into a discussion about my work with AIDS patients from the very beginning of the epidemic, but I wasn't emotionally prepared. On so many levels the subject pained me, and I wanted to avoid it, if only for two weeks. But eight thousand miles from Chicago and my patients, AIDS shadowed me. I could never really escape it. It wasn't just the conversation with the managers of a safari camp.

Two years earlier, while in the Seattle airport waiting to fly to Thailand and then India, we noticed a thin older woman performing calisthenics on the floor of the passenger lounge, in front of two hundred people. Ten days later, in Rajasthan in northern India, this woman and her husband not only were on the same train we took but occupied a room in the same car. She wasn't crazy; she was a restless soul. Her son, who'd traveled extensively in India, had died of AIDS a year earlier. She and her husband were retracing the steps of his spiritual journey before his death and scattering his ashes. How extraordinary, I thought. I viewed our convergence with this couple as merely a coincidence; other people, including Gavin, saw something more cosmic or teleological.

Now, on this same trip to Botswana, we learned of the death of Freddie Mercury, the British rock star—whom, as a classical music snob, I'd never heard of. But at that moment it didn't matter. Here was someone famous who had died of AIDS. Although Mercury was an Indian Parsi, Africa embraced him because he'd been born in Zanzibar. Like so many gay celebrities at the time, Mercury was described as bisexual, which somehow made his death from AIDS more palatable to the public, or at least to his publicist. The revelation grabbed the world's attention. I marveled at his bravery. He could have instructed those closest to him to lie about his diagnosis. Instead his posthumous admission increased sympathy for those afflicted by HIV.

And then, on our way back to camp from a safari one late afternoon, a small bird called a carmine bee-eater hounded our Land Rover. For several miles it swooped, swerved, and wove from one side of the car to the other. At first I was terrified—Alfred Hitchcock's horror film *The Birds* conjured images of pecked-out eyes and seagulls running amok—but our guide explained that vehicles stirred up grasshoppers and other insects in the brush. Bee-eaters usually fly in flocks; this one hunted alone, hovering persistently close to us.

"Can you believe Neal's been dead four months?" Gavin asked, tears welling up. Neal, my former college roommate and confidant, had died in July in Honolulu. Gavin, his thinning blond hair whipped into a frenzy by the wind, turned his attention once again to the bird. The canvas roof of the vehicle had been detached and the windows were rolled down on all sides, giving us a panoramic view of the scrubby landscape as if we were in a boat and not an automobile.

"No, I can't," I said. "Sometimes I don't believe he's really dead. I just think he's gone off somewhere and not called us, that we'll talk to him again someday."

"Maybe he's not dead," Gavin said, motioning toward the bird with a flick of his head. I looked back and smiled uncomfortably at the undulating form that glinted vermilion in the sunlight. Gavin could sometimes joke at an inopportune time. But he had a superstitious side that strained my credulity and sometimes exasperated me. Lately he was beginning to believe in celestial signs and the power of crystals, which was more than I could bear.

"Come on," I said. "That's ridiculous."

"No it isn't," he said forcefully. "I sometimes believe in these things."

"I know you do, but I don't. I don't understand how you can."

"It might do you some good if you started believing in them," he said in a huff.

Had we not been in a Land Rover piloted by a stranger, we might have had a real blow-up. As with so many arguments, it was the subtext that mattered. Gavin never thought that I'd believe Neal's soul inhabited a bee-eater. It was my dismissiveness that irked him. That tendency—the elevation of my convictions over his—irritated him as much as his less rational side irritated me. But despite our disagreement, we were both spooked. Retreating into our internal worlds, we reflected on the bird's significance in silence until we reached camp.

A neighbor had found Neal dead in his apartment and notified his parents, who flew from California to gather up his belongings and arrange for a funeral. His mother called me. It had taken her forever to find my number, she said; the apartment was a mess, with papers, clothes, and scraps of food scattered everywhere. Although Neal dressed meticulously, even ironing his T-shirts, he had no patience for housework. The call caught me by surprise. His mother, whom I'd met only once long before this, asked me about the circumstances of his death, speaking more like an investigator than a distraught mother. I had no idea, I said, feeling like an accomplice to a crime. He'd tried to hide his illness from all of us, including me, his closest friend. The previous year he hadn't returned my telephone calls for weeks, until he revealed that he'd been hospitalized for "pancreatitis"—although he declined to describe his symptoms—and had been discharged on nutrition administered through a large vein in his upper chest. He refused to let me come help take care of him and wouldn't discuss his condition, but the underlying diagnosis was obvious to me. He'd led a promiscuous sex life and had worried about AIDS from the onset of the epidemic.

Neal's loss was so great that it didn't register with me at first. He was one of a handful of people with whom I could be completely honest about my life. Such friendships are rare, take years to build, and usually begin before you're paired with a life partner, who may either accept or feel threatened by the relationship. You grow up together, like siblings, and support each other in the formative years when the future excites and frightens you with its possibilities and tough choices. Every medical school Neal applied to had clamored for him. Unable to tear himself away from California, he turned down Harvard and other Ivy Leagues for the University of California at San Francisco.

Even though we lived thousands of miles apart, we remained close. Gavin and I visited him on several occasions. Showing us sides of Honolulu far from Diamond Head and the white-sand beaches overdeveloped with glitzy hotels and overcrowded with big-bellied tourists, he introduced us to the friendly gay bars and hole-in-the-wall restaurants that served the local fare, a delectable amalgamation of Polynesian, Asian, and European cuisines. The intersection of civilizations fascinated him, for he himself was an intersection of cultures—white, black, and Native American. That fascination rubbed off on me and spurred me to travel the world. He loved the local lingo, in which children were referred to as *keiki*s (pronounced cake-eez) and half-whites *hapa-haoles*. He stayed with us in Chicago once or twice too. The lakefront, with its cement beaches and blissful sunbathers, amused him; and he was unexpectedly chilled to the bone during a jog through Lincoln Park when the temperature dropped thirty degrees in the space of an hour.

But it was the miracle of the telephone that kept our relationship alive. We coached each other through the tedium of the first two years of medical school, when the coursework seemed at times to have little relevance to the careers we envisioned. And while in practice, we exchanged stories about our patients or peers and consulted each other if stumped by a difficult case, though he grew silent and pensive when I described a patient struggling with AIDS, as I often did.

Despite his gregariousness, Neal was a loner. He preferred to remain single and rarely slept with the same man twice; had few friends in Hawaii, where he worked as a psychiatrist at a state hospital, after leaving the death-haunted streets of San Francisco; and moved far from his dearest friends and family. He lived like a refugee, as he put it, ready to move at a moment's notice, with no ties to any person or place. Home wasn't the oasis for him that it was for me, a refuge from a stressful job and a world that hated gay men for their lifestyle, as if lechery defined us and the latest fashions enraptured us. He collected no art, furnished his apartment with cheap furniture, and dressed simply in T-shirts, jeans, or shorts. Even a plant seemed burdensome to him. I thought this lack of attachment to material things was rooted in his vagabond childhood, when he and his family moved every few years to a different continent because his father served in the US Air Force—but on reflection, I realized that he expected to die young. What excites most of us and gives us a reason for existence seemed pointless to Neal.

The thought of Neal in his final weeks, trapped at home, perhaps unable to eat and possibly in pain, unsettled me. How terrible to die alone, to be discovered days or weeks later only because of the stench. I wished he had reached out to me. In addition to grieving his disappearance from my life, I felt hurt, even angry with him. Out of shame, pride, fear, or stubbornness, or perhaps a combination, he had walled himself off from me, even at the end when the wall no longer mattered. I wondered if he had overdosed on narcotics, but I think he would have left a note, if not to me, at least to his parents and two younger brothers. The circumstances of his death would have to remain a mystery.

Now as we bumped along an unpaved road in the Okavango Delta, I tried to dismiss the sadness that overwhelmed me. Neal and I would never grow old together, I thought, sharing our experiences, searching for insights into the mysteries of human existence through another's eyes. He would forever remain for me the young

Neal, frozen as in the photograph that still sits on my bookshelf, a talisman of my past. Decades later his husky voice sometimes intrudes in my mind, in the tone of a philosopher of our young adulthood. The words might remain unclear, but the tone, the spirit, the warmth behind them still resonate. I'd love to mine those tangles of neurons and synapses where so much forgotten remains embedded, if only to return to consciousness the pleasures of our precious friendship.

I couldn't shake the image of the bold red bird and Gavin's superstitious connection of it to Neal. Death was everywhere and unavoidable in Africa—vultures picking clean the stinking carcass of a zebra; the eerie cackles of hyenas as they surrounded, took down, and ripped apart an old cape buffalo; lions roaring over a kill. And then there was the fact that AIDS had started in a remote village in the western part of the continent decades earlier before spreading locally, crossing the oceans, and sweeping around the world, decimating vulnerable populations, gay and straight.

With those morbid thoughts in mind, in December 1991, shortly after I returned to Chicago and the frontlines of a war, I was inspired to write in my journal.

I witness the death struggle very day. Unable to intervene, I watch the beast stalk its victims and feel the pain as it sinks its teeth into its thrashing target, as if I were the target myself. The malevolent hunter haunts me. I fear its footsteps in the night and listen for any signs that it's pursuing me, as if it were outside my tent, calculating how best to reach me, penetrating the thin membrane that separates me from it, finally dragging me out screaming from the feeble defense of sheets and blankets covering my naked body. This is the fascination we have with the great hunters, like the lion, leopard, and cheetah. We identify with both predator and prey, for we can assume both roles. Though in many ways superior, we're not invulnerable. Sometimes our enemies are invisible to the unaided eye, but as malevolent; or they come disguised in our own persona. We become our own stalkers: predator and prey within the same body, a projection of our fears upon ourselves.

: 9 :

Unstoppable Wildfire

(1991–92)

One morning, my Botswanan adventure a receding memory, I received a phone call midway through my exercise routine. I grumbled with annoyance, thinking that I'd had another admission to the hospital; but it was my junior partner C., who in a somber voice let me know that my twenty-three-year-old patient Henry had died an hour earlier. I'd not yet worked up a good sweat and wasn't audibly out of breath—C. wouldn't have known that I'd been exercising. Although I feigned surprise, I couldn't feign sorrow. Another death from AIDS—by now so commonplace for me that a week without a death was an anomaly. One of the commissioners at the Chicago Board of Health, in a backhanded compliment, informed me in 1992 that no one had signed more death certificates in Chicago than I had. That grim statistic sank into some dark hole of my consciousness during the day, surfacing at the most vulnerable moment, in the middle of the night, when sleeplessness unknitted the tightly woven sleeve of care.

I stuffed the news of Henry's death down another dark hole, thanked C., hung up, and returned to the rowing machine. During my tedious routine I always tuned the radio to the local classical music station. The phone call had interrupted one of my favorite pieces of music, a Schubert impromptu. I had half-listened to the dexterous pianist during the conversation, which seemed endless but lasted only thirty seconds. To the beat of the spirited music I now rowed harder, hoping to push up my heart rate, no longer thinking about the patient, his lover, family, or my distraught partner.

How is it that I can be so unmoved? I reflected in a journal entry that evening. *[Henry's] death was routine, as commonplace as another fire or a street murder or a theft. I shouldn't say I didn't react. It took an effort not to react. I felt a certain pressure against my emotions; the pressure was light. It didn't take much to keep the lid on.*

My callousness reminded me of a vignette Tom had once related to me. One of his patients with advanced AIDS had bled into his brain and was on life support in the ICU. Without surgical evacuation of the blood clot, he would die. Uncertain what to do—continue aggressive treatment despite a hopeless prognosis or shift to comfort measures and allow him to die peacefully—Tom called the closest person to this patient, his mother, for guidance. She was about to leave her house to go to the golf course. "Can you call me later, after the game?" she asked.

I was no less indifferent than that woman, I thought. In medicine, emotion is the enemy of clinical judgment. My mentors had taught me, perhaps too well, to suppress those emotions during the critical decision making process. That emotional flatness or tended to my immediate response to another death. But suppression didn't equal extinction. According to the Third Law of Motion, every action results in an equal and opposite reaction. Suppressed emotions have to go somewhere. Instead of sinking into a paralyzing depression over the tragic deaths of all these young men, I sublimated my despair in different ways, not all of which were healthy or conscious, deliberative or rational.

Rushing out of the house early one morning, I forgot my sandwich, which I remembered halfway to the hospital. I didn't have time to turn back or return home later to pick it up. I felt frustrated with myself. Gritting my teeth in anger, I cursed my stupidity. All sorts of negative judgments about my character assailed me. As I went through a list of my deficiencies, a jolt of rage electrified me, and with one hand gripping the steering wheel I slapped myself hard on the face with the other. It wasn't like in the movies when someone smacks a person in the grips of hysteria. My slap was a punishment for a litany of transgressions, imaginary or real — a doctor who failed his patients; son who deceived his parents; gay man who bemoaned his homosexuality: in short, someone who disappointed everyone because of his flaws. I was startled, as if an unexpected assailant had assaulted me. I almost cried, not from pain but from pent-up emotion, but I fought back the tears and chastised myself for such an impulsive gesture.

The heat of the sting subsided, and the fiery red handprint on my left cheek faded into a blush. I glanced in the rearview mirror and wondered if I'd been observed. No one crashed their car or honked at me; passersby hurried to work without pause; I'd not caused any perturbation in the universe. I calmed down, the rage passed, I felt embarrassed and foolish. And then the sensible response came to me: *I'll eat something else, like fruit, from the hospital cafeteria.*

What is it all about? I asked myself later when recording the incident in my journal. *Why such lack of self-control? I can't even tell the psychiatrist about this — It's too shameful. How I treat myself.*

I'd started seeing a psychiatrist in 1989 at the insistence of Gavin, who worried about my constant state of anxiety. At the time I served on the board of Howard Brown, which was in the midst of a financial crisis brought about by AIDS: the number of new STI cases had plummeted, and the clinic's primary revenue stream slowed to a trickle. Its future as a viable institution was uncertain. Members of the board, who realized that the clinic had to branch out in order to survive, took over management of day-to-day operations after the executive director resigned. No one wanted this pillar of the Chicago gay community to fail in the face of an existential threat. But to keep the clinic afloat required hours of extra time on top of our full-time jobs. Moreover, I found it impossible to dedicate time to other organizations, critically important as they were, like ACT-UP (AIDS Coalition to Unleash Power), Open Hand, which provided meals for homebound HIV patients, or Test Positive Aware Network (TPAN), a local grassroots AIDS outreach organization. I couldn't be a doctor caring for hundreds of HIV-infected patients *and* an activist protesting in the streets or lobbying politicians. Of course I had great respect for these organizations, which galvanized the gay community around issues of social justice and the need for access to potentially life-saving treatments. A good number of the leaders and participants were my patients. Still, I had to choose my battles. Treating patients was my greatest strength.

Not long afterward, the stress brought on by the conflict between my desire to please or not disappoint others and my personal, more selfish needs precipitated an episode of atrial fibrillation, an abnormal rhythm disturbance of the heart, which sent me to St. Joe's as a patient. My receptionist cried when she heard that I was in the emergency room. But I hadn't had a heart attack, and I was discharged a few hours later after medication restored the rhythm to normal.

After two years of twice-monthly visits with Dr. D., I wasn't really better off psychologically. For that I blame myself more than I blame him—he was sympathetic, kind, and insightful. I still hadn't developed a level of trust that would have allowed me tell him about the slap. It would have been the perfect talking point, but I chickened out. I hadn't reached rock bottom. Like an alcoholic who isn't ready to give up drink, I wasn't ready to let down my guard sufficiently to expose the shame that lay at the heart of my insecurities and fueled my anxiety. I'm a highly defended person, to use psychotherapeutic lingo. To tear down those thick, high walls protecting a vulnerable core would take decades.

Perhaps I would have kept hacking away at it, but Dr. D. moved to California. His departure provided the perfect excuse to halt the laborious, painful, and often frustrating process of psychotherapy.

Instead of exploring the deeper meaning behind my self-punishment with Dr. D., I dismissed the slap as something minor, like tripping on the sidewalk or slipping on the ice. No harm had come—I didn't develop a black eye, break a jaw, or knock out a tooth. Besides, I had too much else on my mind that morning. The day was busy like most days: mortally ill people I couldn't save, morning report with burned-out nurses, a trip to the office in congested traffic, phone messages requiring more than yes and no answers, frightened but not yet mortally ill patients in my waiting room and exam rooms. a return to the hospital to attend a depressing lecture, "AIDS and the Heart," at noon. back to the office, more phone calls, packed afternoon schedule. For twelve hours I had no break, or brakes. Go, go, go, go, go. Like a locomotive hurtling down a track, I would halt only if derailed. It would take more than a slap to derail me, but what that would be I didn't know and hoped never to find out.

––––––

It's a cold, blustery day in late December 1991, the wind bone-chilling, the skies gray. The tan from my trip to Botswana is fading. I enter the hospital, head for the doctor's lounge, and punch my private code on the computer key board to generate my list of patients. Still bundled up in my down jacket, I go to my mailbox and sort through the mail, which includes lab results, notes from the emergency department, and other papers. Then I exchange my parka for my gray coat and take the elevator to the third-floor radiology department. One of the clerks thanks me for the white poinsettia I'd brought to her and her fellow clerks in gratitude for their excellent service. Usually reserved, she is loquacious and seems genuinely pleased. She talks about how she has to stop eating Christmas chocolates because she's getting too fat. The plant with its ivory petals is on a cabinet, brightening the dreary file room with its array of folders containing x-rays. Cheerfully, she searches for an x-ray that appears to be missing. She's so nice, I can't be upset and spoil the moment with a tantrum. With a sigh, I leave and take the elevator to 11 West, where I peruse my patients' charts at the nurses' station, which is surprisingly quiet. Someone has decorated the unit with red stockings hanging from the ceiling. The hallway is snowing socks.

Bob J. is the first person I visit. His curtain is drawn, separating him from his roommate. He is in a reclining chair, feet elevated, all smiles when he sees me. Seated in profile beside him fussing with his intravenous line is one of the nurses, whom he shoos away.

"Get over here, I'm talking to you first," he says to me.

Bob has one of those expressive faces that make me want to

laugh. Always upbeat, he puts me in good spirits. He has bright, dancing green eyes, black hair artificially curled, and ruddy, chubby cheeks. Although not handsome, he has a winning personality. A purplish KS lesion that once bubbled up on his upper lip has faded to a stain.

"I look like Madonna," he says, referring to the lesion on his pooched lip as if it were a birthmark. "I feel great. Send me home."

His dangerously low white blood count—the reason for his admission to the hospital—has improved with a new medication called Neupogen, a bone marrow stimulant that has revolutionized the treatment of many cancers. Chemotherapy suppresses the cells that fight off infections. Neupogen counteracts that effect and allows doctors to be more aggressive with cancer-fighting agents, thus increasing the chances for survival. Although in the case of AIDS, it is only delaying the inevitable.

Down the hall from Bob is Manny, who is engrossed in a phone conversation. First I see his roommate, Alex, who is bundled up to his neck in blankets, his face with purple-splotched nose exposed. He has beautiful eyes framed by thick lashes and is the vision of a sick person, absent a thermometer in his mouth and water bottle on his head. A man of few words, he exudes depression, although he denies feeling depressed. Because he hardly speaks, he looks melancholic yet doesn't seem to grasp the enormity of his situation, like a child during a bombing raid who plays with toys despite the all-encompassing danger. He tells me that he feels better, that he's eating well. He still requires nutrition pumped through his veins to combat malabsorption from unrelenting diarrhea, which has diminished but not ended. His fevers have abated, and with luck he may be able to go home soon.

I return to Manny, who has gotten off the phone. His situation is complicated by the fact that he's married with children and has lived a secret gay life. For months I implored him to stop having sex with his wife, but to no avail. I agonized about what to do and sought counsel from Tom and Gavin, who were both as uncertain as I. I contemplated notifying the police or the Board of Health but worried about the potential breach in patient confidentiality. In anticipation of the fallout—breach of confidentiality or failure to notify a person at risk—I even considered contacting my malpractice carrier to warn of a potential lawsuit, either from Manny or from Manny's wife, depending. I consulted an ethicist, but our conversations ended inconclusively. I'd never confronted such a moral dilemma before in my career and felt woefully inept in dealing with it. I rued my lack of training as a legal expert or philosopher.

After Manny's AIDS diagnosis, his wife tested positive for HIV. For weeks she sobbed uncontrollably, and nothing I said consoled her. Her situation is too painful for me to contemplate: a mother, the wife of a dying husband, and herself possibly dying. I wonder what will become of their children. This is a scenario from a country torn by war, not something commonly experienced in the United States except in the era of slavery.

A few years earlier I'd taken care of a man named Orlando, a janitor in a Catholic church who died of AIDS in 1986, leaving behind a wife and two sons aged ten and twelve. Six months later his wife, who was HIV negative, died unexpectedly of a brain aneurysm. The only relatives lived in Colombia and Mexico. A deacon at the church, a close friend of Orlando, took custody of the boys. Amazingly, Orlando had had the foresight to obtain life insurance shortly before his AIDS diagnosis. Yet the adjudicator from the insurance company chose to deny the disbursement of money to the children on the grounds that Orlando had lied not about his HIV status but about smoking, which had nothing to do with his death. At his own expense, the deacon hired the best attorney he could find and got the decision overruled by a judge. A gay man himself with no experience as a parent, the deacon became de facto father and is successfully raising the boys into adulthood. I can only hope that an equally loving benefactor will be found for Manny's soon-to-be-orphaned children.

Manny is curled up toward the wall of his room. I call to him and he rolls over, pulling himself into a sitting position as he elevates the head of the bed. His face has lost its boyish underlying fat, and the slack skin is wrinkled with worry. Accepting the certainty of his death and no longer angry or full of unrealistic expectations, he has withdrawn from the world. With furrowed brow, he looks out at some invisible landmark beyond fear.

"Manny, we can't send you home," I say. "It seems that the hospice people won't help at home unless you tell your kids your diagnosis. They're at risk because they might come in contact with your body fluids. They'll have to know why they need to be careful."

"I can't," he says.

"I know, so you have to stay here. Your wife can't care for you alone. I won't send you home on morphine without support from nurses."

"Fine, I stay here then," he says in his Greek accent.

"You'll have to leave the AIDS unit and go to the skilled unit, a kind of nursing home in the hospital," I say. "They're not as attentive down there because the nurses have more patients to attend to than on the AIDS unit."

"That's OK," he says. "Private room? Good." He brings the phone to his lap. "I call my wife. She want to speak to you. I dunno what."

He presses down hard on each button like a neophyte using a typewriter for the first time. There's frustration in his fingertips. He says something in Greek.

"Here," he says, thrusting the phone at me. I talk to his wife. Her sobs during the last few months have devolved into whimpers, and she speaks in a cracking voice like someone who has cried herself into exhaustion. Despair has sharpened her sense of the world.

"He don't talk to me," she says, her English as awkward English as her husband's. "Guilt?"

As I tell her that he's withdrawing from the world, Manny listens, watching from the corner of his eye.

"He's there listening, isn't he?" she asks. "We talk later about this, OK?"

Manny stares at his feet. His hair is disheveled, and he reminds me of the heavy-lidded *Woman before the Aquarium* by Henri Matisse, a painting at the Art Institute of Chicago. Her chin resting on a forearm, the melancholic woman appears to be gazing at a gold-fish bowl but clearly looks through it or, self-absorbed, doesn't see the bowl at all.

"Doc, I get nightmares," he says. "I think medicine too strong. We turn it down, OK?"

"Yes," I say. "I'll tell the nurse." I get up to leave.

"Thanks for comin'," he says.

During our early encounters I despised him for his carelessness with his wife. Now I feel more sympathetic toward him. Despite his irresponsible behavior, I admire his courage and wonder if I will be as graceful when my death looms. No doubt he infected his wife long before I warned him to protect her—or so I rationalize to let myself off the hook. He didn't purposefully infect her. I'm not even sure he considered himself to be a person at risk, so powerful was the denial. In the 1980s antigay prejudice in the Greek immigrant community and in the United States compelled him to live a double life. In that regard he wasn't much different from many gay men of my generation. There are a good number of Mannys in the world with equally unlucky wives, as proven by the epidemic in sub-Saharan Africa, where AIDS is a heterosexual disease. His life is tragic, not criminal, at least in my opinion. At worst, he is guilty of involuntary manslaughter. And even if he's guilty of more, he'd already been given the worst possible sentence, without the benefit of a judge and jury. I reach out to hug him: *who am I to judge?* I ask. As healers, doctors must suspend judgment and not make choices in determining who shall or shall not be treated. Grateful for my sympathy, Manny embraces me, as if rebuffed and then reaccepted.

"Doc, you're a real friend," he says, half-smiling.

———

On a scale of human suffering, 1992 hardly differed from the previous eleven years of the AIDS crisis. My small triumphs—shifting the curve of death from months to a couple of years because we could now cure several opportunistic infections and prevent their recurrence—ultimately gave way to defeat as my patients died of some other untreatable opportunistic infection or cancer. Yet that shift in the curve signaled progress of a sort. Cancer specialists at the time couldn't boast a similar record of success, if by success we meant putting off death for years instead of months. AIDS patients were living longer, even if we couldn't treat the underlying HIV. I clung to the slimmest of slimmest hope that my patients with AIDS could survive just long enough for medications to cure them or put them into remission.

Nevertheless, it amazed me how swiftly someone could proceed from initial infection to death from AIDS. In the late 1980s one of my patients, a chronically depressed man in his mid-fifties, convinced his reluctant HIV-positive boyfriend to fuck him without a condom. Like a wife who chooses to die on the funeral pyre of her dead husband, he expressed a wish to go down in flames with his lover. I pleaded with him not to be so reckless and pointed out that he had two grown children and a small number of friends who loved him and didn't want him to die. It didn't matter. He was determined to get AIDS. Refusing antidepressants and a referral for psychotherapy, he eventually got what he wanted and died miserably two years later.

Miraculous treatments didn't appear imminent. In July 1991 I went to Florence to attend the Seventh International AIDS Conference, which had nothing to offer but gloom-and-doom predictions of how many more people worldwide would be infected with HIV by 1995. Like an unstoppable wildfire, AIDS swept the globe. HIV was no longer a gay man's disease, except in the United States and Western Europe. Two-thirds of cases in the developing world were in heterosexuals. Every sexually active person not in a monogamous relationship was theoretically at risk of exposure to HIV, a fact that panicked a small cadre of heterosexual patients that showed up in my office obsessed with the idea that they'd contracted HIV, no matter how innocuous their sexual contact with a prostitute or woman picked up in a bar had been. Nothing I said, no reassurance about the impossibility ("a blowjob only?" or "you used a condom?"), no test I performed convinced them. I half-expected an expression of relief if they tested positive. As a self-flagellating person, I understood their obsession. Think the worst: that was my motto. Then you'll be emotionally prepared for a bad diagnosis and prognosis. Yet I wasn't so obsessive that I'd disbelieve evidence to the contrary.

At the Florence conference one researcher, Dr. William Haseltine of Harvard University, described how HIV could invade the body through the mucosal surfaces of the genital and gastrointestinal tracts without trauma or direct entrance into the bloodstream. This reinforced the importance of condom use. It didn't matter if a gay man topped or bottomed; both practices were risky. Dr. Haseltine's research also underscored the difficulty of developing a vaccine, because generating an antibody response cannot by itself control HIV infection. If the body produced effective antibodies against HIV, a vaccine would have been developed in the 1980s, relegating HIV to a footnote of medical history. To stop the spread of AIDS, the only tool we had in 1991, besides screening the blood supply to prevent transmission through transfusions, was selling the idea of safe sex, and that wasn't working.

Florence was an interesting place to hold the conference. More than six hundred years earlier the bubonic plague, or Black Death, made a sudden appearance in the city, decimating its population and forcing those not afflicted to flee to the countryside or hole up in their homes in a vain attempt to escape its ravages.

"Against these maladies the advice of doctors and the power of medicine appeared useless and unavailing," wrote Giovanni Boccaccio in 1353. The same words could have been penned in 1981, at the onset of the AIDS epidemic in the United States. "Perhaps the disease was such that no remedy was possible, or the problem lay with those who were treating it . . . and since none of them had any idea what was causing the disease, they could hardly prescribe an appropriate remedy for it."

"Some of the people were of the opinion that living moderately and being abstemious would really help them resist the disease," Boccaccio continued, as if he were describing the gay community and my patients once we all grasped the existential threat. "Others, holding the contrary opinion, maintained that the surest medicine for such an evil disease was to drink heavily, enjoying life's pleasures, and go about singing and having fun, satisfying their appetites . . . while laughing at everything and turning whatever happened into a joke. . . . There were others who took a middle course between the two." No matter how one responded, the Black Death didn't discriminate.

Deriving little pleasure from the conference, Gavin and I explored the old city's cobblestone streets, majestic churches, and sculptural masterpieces. We crossed the Arno River by way of the Ponte Vecchio, the only bridge from medieval or Renaissance times to have survived aerial bombing during World War II. No visit to Florence would have been complete without viewing Michelangelo's *David*, an idealized representation of young male beauty—with its disappointingly small penis (Michelangelo wasn't a size queen)—not to be missed by any respectable gay man.

Gavin and I weren't the only Chicagoans attending the conference. There was a small contingent of fellow AIDS healthcare providers, and many of us met up afterward like warriors shooting the breeze in a smoky bar, sharing stories and showing off wounds. Tom was there too. In July 1991, five months before Henry's death, we hired another doctor, C., who'd barely settled into his office when Tom and I took off, leaving him alone for five days to manage a practice of staggering complexity. Having worked with us for three years as a family practice resident caring for our hospitalized patients, he was no greenhorn; and our nurse Maureen, as knowledgeable and capable as any doctor, helped. He relished the challenge, he said—but the builders of the Great Pyramid might have said the same thing before laying the first stone. He survived the ordeal but extracted promises from us never to leave him alone again.

After seven years of practice, Tom and I were tired and irritable, sometimes snapping at patients, more often snapping at staff. When a patient with AIDS called me to spout a litany of complaints against one of my nurses, the receptionists, and me, I lashed out, remarking that I was sick of people projecting their frustrations with their own health problems onto others. He fired me, but in six months he called to apologize and begged to return to the practice. I accepted his apology and apologized in return for my intemperance.

Every other week Tom and I had taken call, and we covered for each other when one of us went out of town. Taking call meant interruptions while at dinner or a concert, in the middle of the night, or at any time during the weekend. In the concert hall or opera house we vied for access to the pay phone during intermission, mindful of the clock, the time crunch threatening to ruin the evening's enjoyment. When paged while on errands, I hunted for the nearest phone booth and hoped I could find a parking space without getting a ticket. And after returning from a vacation we'd have to make up for the time by taking call for two or three weeks in a row, which left us questioning whether it was worth leaving town for more than twenty-four hours.

There were nights when I got little sleep because the phone rang or pager beeped multiple times, at first from a frantic ill patient, followed by the ER doctor when that patient showed up for evaluation, and hours later from the intern or resident after admitting him. And the patient could be one of several admissions. I'm a poor sleeper. If I expect a phone call or page, I lie in bed full of anxiety, unable to sleep—will it be midnight, 1:00 a.m., 2:00 a.m., or later before my phone shrieks or pager reverberates like a high-pitched drill? If I somehow do drift off to sleep, later I won't be able to fall back asleep after discussing the details of the case because of the rush of adrenaline. It was worse than being an intern and resident—at least those years had time limits. This was the life of a doctor, of course; but in a war there are more casualties than during peacetime. The war against AIDS appeared to have no time limit; the prospect of sleep, I absurdly thought, would have to wait until my death. Tom and I desperately needed a third partner to give us time to recuperate, and to continue to absorb the increasing number of patients flocking to our practice like refugees.

Gavin's call schedule did not always dovetail with mine. There were times when I would be on call but he wasn't or vice versa. When I was paged, he woke up too. In a huff, he would pull the blankets over his head. When the shoe was on the other foot, more than once I growled at him for not moving to the bathroom out of earshot instead of talking, even yelling when frustrated, on the chaise longue a few steps from our bed. He relaxed there as if on a beach chair, left ankle crossed over his right knee, head hanging over an arm as he gesticulated with a free hand. The bedroom in our house in Bucktown was capacious, with twelve-foot ceilings and thick curtains hiding a wall of windows, which amplified Gavin's voice as if in an amphitheater. The image of him on the chaise is funny to me now. It wasn't then.

———

Gavin and I had moved to Bucktown in February 1991 because we were tired of the politics of a condominium association. We wanted a free-standing home we could afford in the city. Bucktown had seen better days, and a number of oldtimers, mainly people of Polish or Ukrainian descent, still occupied some of the houses. In the 1960s, when many white families like my own had fled the city for the suburbs, ostensibly for a better education for their children, Bucktown declined and buildings were abandoned. Poor families (mainly Hispanics) and artists moved in, followed by developers. In its crumbling state, Bucktown had charm. Funky restaurants doubling as art galleries had sprung up; Gavin and I were amused to be the two square people in a space where everyone else had multicolored hair, paint on their fingers, tattoos on exposed skin, and nose rings. One acquaintance in Bucktown who out of curiosity posted a sign inviting anyone gay in the area to his house for a party was surprised that more than a hundred people showed up, which was refreshing. Boys' Town no longer had a monopoly on gay life in Chicago, if it ever had.

Our three-story brick and glass house didn't resemble the A-frames, bungalows, or brownstones around it. The first floor sat sunken halfway below street level and was set back to permit a small front garden. For privacy and protection, an elegant wrought-iron fence enclosed the property. At the top of the facade the architect had appended whimsical flourishes, a central cement half-circle flanked on each corner by a pyramid. A skylight and glass block on one wall of the dining room made the interior light and airy. It was love at first sight for me; Gavin needed convincing because even in an up-and-coming neighborhood, the list price stretched our budget. A similar house on the Gold Coast would have cost two or three times as much.

When I showed the house to my parents, my mother reacted with skepticism and my father kept his thoughts to himself.

"It's a beautiful house," I said defensively.

"Yes, it is," she agreed.

"It's only about two miles west of my office near Cabrini Green, and it's an easy drive to your house in Wilmette," I rationalized.

"But look at the neighborhood," she pointed out, like a dentist noting that one good tooth beside a row of rotting ones didn't brighten the smile.

One Saturday afternoon that first fall, I was in the front garden planting tulips. As I squatted in the dirt digging six-inch holes, inserting a papery bulb into each one, and adding fertilizer before burying it, I heard a distant popping sound. I stopped and stood up to listen with ears twitching forward and fine hairs on my neck standing upright like those of a stalked animal. No one else seemed perturbed. Children on a nearby street didn't cease playing. Our three-month-old puppy Monty dashed around the yard throwing up dirt as he ran in circles. Like a fever heralding the onset of a dangerous illness, the pops portended something ominous to me. As I was about to resume my gardening, shooing Monty away, I looked up and observed a young man slinking by my fence, glancing behind him and paying no attention to me. Later I noticed a trail of blood along the fence line. Within minutes, hysterical screams emanated from a nearby house.

"He's been shot, he's been shot!" someone cried.

I grabbed Monty and asked myself, *What should I do? Should I shout "I'm a doctor" and rush to help? Should I call the police? Should I lock myself in the house and hide from any stray bullets?*

Before I could make a decision, a car with big wheels pulled up, the wounded teenager was shoved inside, and the driver raced away, hopefully to a hospital, leaving me to ponder the severity of the boy's injury. And like a pond whose surface has been disturbed by the toss of a stone and then returns to placidity, life went on as if nothing significant had happened. The children continued to play, old ladies strolled by with their pushcarts, and I finished planting. But the incident unnerved me. What kind of neighborhood was this? Moreover, had I been cowardly, equivocating rather than thrusting myself into a potentially dangerous situation, concerned more about my life than about that of the wounded boy?

When it came to AIDS patients, however, I didn't equivocate. I never shunned an AIDS patient or hesitated to treat someone because of fear for my own health or safety. There were times when I put myself in harm's way. In the earliest days of the epidemic, when we didn't know if AIDS, like the Ebola virus, could be transmitted through sweat, saliva, or other bodily secretions besides blood, I often hugged my patients to reassure them that they weren't "lepers," as they often referred to themselves. Because of my habit of sitting on the side of a patient's bed, holding his hand as we talked, I've even sat on urine-soaked sheets. Once when I was drawing blood on a patient with HIV, the seal around the needle in a syringe broke and blood leaked onto my ungloved hand. We looked at each other in stunned silence. That was in the mid-1980s, before the CDC issued the policy of universal precautions in which everyone should wear gloves and protective eyewear or a mask when dealing with potentially infectious body fluids. Later I stuck myself several times while performing a procedure in the office, like draining an abscess, performing a spinal tap, or taking a biopsy of a skin lesion. Each time I panicked a bit, but I didn't get infected.

Now and then I felt physically threatened as the bearer of bad news. The boyfriend of a patient who'd failed all treatments for PCP, including an experimental one, ambushed me one morning during rounds. Furious that his lover was dying, he came up from behind, fist raised as if to punch me, rage in his eyes, but I defused the situation by reminding him that we were all on the same side. I wanted his partner to get better just like he did, and was doing everything in my power to rid him of PCP, but I couldn't restore the health of his immune system. The virus was the enemy, I said, not me. He broke down in tears and we embraced.

That moment, sometime in 1990 or 1991, seemed like a revelation to me because I spoke the truth: the virus was the enemy, not I. I could forgive myself, I thought, for losing patients to this dreadful disease; their deaths were not my fault. Yet that revelation provided no consolation for me. It didn't make the losses less dreadful or depressing, nor did it make my days brighter or nights less tortured.

: 10 :

Dead Men Walking

(1992)

Bill was my final patient that day. It was a Tuesday in February 1992, one of my late nights when I finished seeing patients at the office at 7:00 p.m. When I entered the examination room, he was sitting on the bulky leather table leaning against the wall, the picture of despair. Already weary after a twelve-hour day, at that depressing image I felt as if I were a deflating balloon, but I did my best to appear fresh and interested. His mother and his lover David, who was also one of my patients, sat facing me. They were all pale, but for different reasons: Bill, who was gaunt, anemic, wasting away, skeletal and dying of AIDS; David, Italian, robust, chubby, and balding, with unblemished olive skin and large imploring, frightened brown eyes; and Bill's mother, a quiet and reticent lady with pale skin and a likeness to her son—the same blue eyes, a "lantern jaw," her lower lip tucked beneath the upper one.

Bill had once been stoic, but by this stage in his illness he tended to become strident. With each complaint his voice rose into a high tenor and then, as if overcome by the force of his feelings, dropped into a lower register as he collapsed into hopelessness and despair. The preceding weeks hadn't been good for him. After he developed numbness and weakness of the left side of his body, I'd ordered a brain scan. The scan showed multiple round tumors whose edges lit up like rings with contrast material. At first I thought he had toxoplasmosis, a once-rare infection picked up from cats or from eating raw meat that had become common since the onset of the AIDS epidemic. Although a screening blood test for the infection was negative, I put him on medications for it anyway. After only one week he stopped them because of intolerable side effects, mainly intractable diarrhea and stool incontinence. The next step was to try something experimental, but I needed a definitive diagnosis before applying for it through an expanded access program. That program, sanctioned by the Food and Drug Administration at the urging of AIDS activists, permitted the use of promising medications in life-threatening situations before their ultimate approval and marketing. The application process wasn't onerous, and if the patient was approved he received the drug free of charge.

To get a definitive diagnosis, I needed a brain biopsy. Bill reluctantly agreed, but the process leading up to the biopsy had turned into a small fiasco. I consulted a neurosurgeon, who scheduled the biopsy, but his nurse ordered the wrong preoperative laboratory tests. Moreover, when Bill showed up for the blood draw, no one had any orders at all and he was redirected to the admitting office for clarification. Someone had ordered an EKG and chest x-ray. Bill protested their necessity. The clerk dismissed his protests. Telephoning me in anger, Bill accused everyone of incompetence and lack of caring. He hadn't even met the neurosurgeon and no longer wanted the biopsy.

"No one listens to me!" he exclaimed.

The brain biopsy frightened Bill, as it would frighten anyone, because the brain isn't an organ that can regenerate. Any damage to it is permanent and irreversible. Normally such a procedure, although scary in concept, was uneventful and didn't require admission to the hospital, because complications were rare and the amount of material collected was minuscule. But our arrangements looked sloppy and seemed to forebode disaster. When consoling and reassuring Bill didn't work, I suggested delaying the procedure because I didn't want him to have a biopsy if he felt angry, frustrated, or afraid. I also hadn't forgotten that he was a lawyer. After a half hour of pushing and pulling, he again agreed to undergo the procedure. We did need one more test, I told him, which could only be performed at the hospital. Taking personal responsibility for ensuring smoothness and accuracy, I scheduled the test myself and promised to call him twenty-four hours afterward to give him the results, which I did. I had regained his confidence.

The day after the biopsy itself, he called to inform me that he'd developed sudden weakness of his left hand immediately after the biopsy, which didn't seem possible to me because the sample was taken from a site nowhere near the area of his brain controlling muscle function. When I spoke to him a couple of days later, he said he was worse. I didn't have good news for him: the biopsy didn't show toxoplasmosis. The result was helpful only because it narrowed the possibilities to untreatable conditions.

These were the circumstances that had led to that early evening visit. An aura of sadness filled the room, as there usually is in this kind of situation. I began by recapping Bill's recent medical history, mostly for his mother's sake. In November 1991 Bill had developed CMV retinitis and lost a lot of weight, but with treatment he recovered some of his vision and weight. In January when he complained of numbness on the left side of his body, a brain scan proved abnormal, which is what ultimately led to the brain biopsy. His mother nodded now and then as if understanding my words, though she showed little emotion. It was hard for me to know what she was really feeling. I spoke as simply as possible, defining my terms. I glanced over to Bill, who sat with drooping shoulders against the wall, squinting behind glasses with a mixture of pain and annoyance. Occasionally he sighed. David's eyes were wide and doelike. He leaned forward, clutching Bill's coat. I explained that even if we could treat Bill's current problem, something would eventually happen that wasn't treatable.

And then I moved on to the part of the conversation that was inevitable when speaking to the families of a terminally ill patient: what to do next. In the process of death and dying, patients follow Elizabeth Kubler-Ross's five-stage algorithm, although always shifting among levels not in clearly delineated steps but in a two-step-forward, one-step-back pattern. So do the relatives, but often they're out of step with the patient or the doctor. Those five stages are shock, denial, anger, bargaining, and acceptance. David was in the bargaining stage; Bill was on the verge of acceptance; his mother—I wasn't sure. David asked if there were any other therapies available. What about intravenous Vitamin C or anything else? Should Bill see a neurologist? Who was the best neurologist in Chicago? Should he go to New York City or San Francisco? Bill's mother nodded passively.

"What about my hand, my hand?" Bill asked sharply. "I can't move it. It got worse right after the surgery."

Really? I thought. In my mind it was a progressive problem, not sudden in onset—a result of whatever was causing the lesions in his brain.

Sighing with disgust, Bill said, "I told you. No one ever listens!"

But he wasn't as forceful as he might have been. He was full of despair, which blunted his anger. I choked on my words and felt my cheeks grow hot. Was I blushing? I cursed my lack of control over my autonomic nervous system. How was I to save face? Did I need to save face? Was I going to be sued? I'd promised Bill no ill effects from the procedure and then had noted all the problems leading up to the biopsy. *Disaster? No*, I thought, but I felt terrible. There was nothing that could be done about the hand. David and Bill focused on an unfortunate symptom and avoided the bigger picture.

The truth was, Bill was dying and no one wanted to confront this fact. Our conversation circled the issue, though I'd been building up to it. At the critical moment I was again too cautious. I'm generally not direct or blunt when talking about death. I'm like a director who creates the scene and then hopes the characters will appear on cue, ready to play their parts. But usually it turns out to be an in medias res drama, where the characters stumble onto the truth after much pain and many missteps, regardless of the director's earnest efforts. I'm never in as much control as I'd like to be. No matter how much I try to anticipate thoughts, feelings, and expectations, I can't know exactly what goes on in people's hearts. We all have different agendas and different methods for coping with stress. In this instance, I'd hoped that Bill, his mom, or David would bring up the issue of death, but they weren't ready, and my attempt to bring them to that point fell flat.

I offered the name of a nationally recognized expert in AIDS-related neurological diseases, at Northwestern. David conceded that it was Bill's decision, but Bill made no specific comment about my recommendation. I examined him in a cursory manner and noted that his left hand was indeed weak, although he could move the rest of his arm. His left leg was also slightly weak. When I poked him with a pinwheel, his sensation was diminished but not absent on the left side, especially on his left hand and forearm. His knees and arms kicked and jerked symmetrically at the mild pounding of my red rubber reflex hammer. From a neurological perspective the findings made no sense to me, but my knowledge of neurology was fuzzy. I still wondered whether the weakness was some sort of hysterical reaction, something psychological rather than physiological. I didn't want the findings to be real, because if they were they might somehow have occurred as a result of the brain biopsy—a slight amount of swelling in the brain, perhaps.

I prescribed a powerful steroid medication that could reduce swelling in the brain from lesions or trauma. In seventy-two hours we might see improvement, I said, but that wasn't enough for Bill. He wanted to try the experimental medication for toxoplasmosis. I wasn't sure I could get it for him because his tests weren't consistent with toxoplasmosis, but I promised to do my best. The manufacturer might release it based on the brain scan alone, I said.

Thirty emotionally taxing minutes had passed. I felt drained. I asked Bill to call me in three days to report his progress. When I shook his mother's hand, she smiled. Bill hugged me. There was no animosity toward me after all, I thought. He was so thin, fragile, and weak. He smiled at me in his usual fashion, eyes shut, crow's feet on the edges, nose scrunched as if he'd tasted something tart. David looked terrified. Anxiety seemed to course like electricity beneath his smooth, pale olive skin. He too hugged me. They were all desperate, grasping at straws.

I fought off feelings that Gavin described in himself, the sense that Dr. C., the neurologist at Northwestern, would expose me as an impostor. Here I was, an expert in the new field of HIV/AIDS medicine, respected for his knowledge and expertise yet obsessed by irrational, even ludicrous thoughts! As an expert, I'd been accustomed to being the person from whom patients sought second opinions, and now I was being questioned. After all these years second opinions still threatened me, making me doubt my judgment and skills. I could trace the thread of insecurity far back into childhood, when I was a kid in second grade who stood up and cried because a prize had been given to a student who'd performed as well as I.

"You have to let other people win too," my beloved teacher had chided me. She was right, but the decision didn't hurt any less.

Already composing a history and defense of my management with an imaginary Dr. C., I feared being accused of incompetence and criticized for improper care. But what if I'd been wrong not only in my diagnosis but also in my treatment plan? Even though Bill's death was preordained at this point, such an error could have shortened his life by a few precious weeks or months, robbing him of quality time with his lover and mother. I was acutely aware that doctors make mistakes, and sometimes I held myself to standards that were impossibly high: the truth is that sooner or later we all err, sometimes grievously. Surgeons may inadvertently lacerate an organ; nonsurgeons may miss a brewing cancer. Practicing medicine is a balancing act: I had to inspire confidence in my patients while at the same time maintaining a degree of humility and avoiding arrogance. A hint of humility made you more human. I said goodbye, and Bill walked gingerly out of the room with a slight limp, supported on either side by mother and lover.

A few weeks later Bill was back in the hospital. Dr. C. had found nothing amiss in our workup or management and had nothing new to offer. In the meantime Bill had developed fevers, more weakness, and shortness of breath. A blood test showed severe anemia, and I ordered a blood transfusion. A few days later he was extremely short of breath and his lips, fingers, and toes were blue. A chest x-ray revealed pneumonia, and his white blood cell count had dropped to a dangerously low level. Although doses of steroids boosted his energy, his death now seemed imminent.

David urged me not to say anything negative to Bill. Although I obliged, I insisted that David himself have a frank talk with me. He was more resigned to Bill's fate than he'd been four weeks earlier. Could I have helped him more by telling him that his own HIV test one and a half years earlier was negative? He'd never called me, but I couldn't stand it anymore. He almost yelled at me when I started to tell him, but when he heard the news, tears came to his eyes and he embraced me, sobbing. He said that he'd planned to wait until "it was all over with Bill" before calling me to get the results. It wasn't something he could deal with while Bill was alive.

For comfort, I put Bill on a morphine drip. He was also on a number of other medications, including one to treat PCP, for that had recurred despite attempts to prevent it, and two antibiotics to treat other infections that might be brewing but not yet detected. It was a move of desperation. I was casting a wide net in one final attempt to save his life. Through a mask I pumped the maximum amount of oxygen I could give him without placing him on a ventilator. He puffed away, although he was still alert and appeared comfortable. He asked me when he could go home. I told him that he could go when it was obvious that his condition had improved, an answer he accepted. Before I left, he vomited some blood.

Distressed, David wondered if he should remain at Bill's bedside and not go to this office. I urged him to leave in order to get some rest, but he opted to stay. He started to cry again when he told me that Bill's mother was flying in and would take a cab to the hospital. I'm not sure what provoked the tears, except that he was afraid of alarming Bill and conveying the message that the end was near. I doubted Bill would last the night.

When I entered his room at 6:30 the following morning, he was "Cheyne-Stoking," a form of respiration characterized by deep, rapid breaths alternating with periods of shallow breathing or no breathing at all, a sign that his death was imminent. Bill's mother sat on a futon the nurses had brought her; David leaned forward on one of the chairs, bracing his knees with his hands and watching his lover's final gasps. It had been a bad night. To make Bill more comfortable, the head of his bed had been elevated at a 45-degree angle, but he looked anything but comfortable. His head was cocked at an awkward angle, and his chin rested on his right shoulder while his arms hung limply at his sides. His face had a waxlike quality, the taut skin outlining the underlying bone. I lifted the lid of one of his partially open eyes and noted a fixed and dilated pupil, another sign of impending death. The only sound in the room was his waxing and waning breaths, amplified by the oxygen mask. When I called his name, he didn't respond, nor did I elicit any reaction as I dug a knuckle into his sternum—a maneuver that might seem cruel but is meant to assess the level of consciousness and degree of brain damage. I picked up the covers and moved his legs, which were as flaccid as those of a rag doll. His heartbeat remained surprisingly strong.

I motioned to Bill's mother and David, and we walked across the hall to the lounge. It's my practice not to have difficult conversations in front of a comatose patient. One never knows what he can hear or understand, though now that his pupils were fixed and dilated, Bill's higher cognitive functioning had ceased and he would have heard or understood nothing. I also don't believe in telling the patient one thing, the family another. During a telephone conversation earlier, Bill's mother had expressed concern that David was still in denial about her son's illness. David kept talking as if there was still hope, she said. I explained to her that everyone reaches acceptance at different rates.

The filthy state of the lounge on 11 West embarrassed me. The air was thick with cigarette smoke. Ashes and bits of food soiled the table. Someone had forgotten to turn off the television. I turned it off. The three of us sat down and reviewed Bill's current condition. Things looked ominous, I said. The conversation continued along these lines for a few minutes before David instinctively got up and rushed to Bill's side. Moments later he motioned to us.

"I think he's dead," he said.

When I entered the room, Bill's position hadn't changed, but the Cheyne-Stoke breathing had ceased and his mouth hung open without a twitch or quiver. I took my time examining him, putting my fingers on his cooling wrist to feel for a pulse and then shining a light into, away from, into, and away from his glazed eyes until I was satisfied that they didn't react. I removed the ophthalmoscope from its perch on the wall above the headboard and bent downward, my nose almost touching his waxy gray cheek as I peered into both retinas to look for the telltale signs of the cessation of active circulation. As I slowly drew back, I removed my stethoscope from a side pocket, slipped its earpieces into my ears, and pressed the bell onto the left side of his chest, listening for a couple of minutes. It was like being inside a shell, the outside world blocked out almost completely, my own breathing all that I could hear. When I couldn't detect heart sounds, I stood up and let the earpieces slide down around my neck. It was at this point that I pronounced him dead.

Bill's mother sobbed uncontrollably, her head bent toward her chest and hands raised to her temples. David looked stunned but remained in control of his emotions. Bill's mother's tears brought tears to my own eyes. During the last few months I'd become fond of her. Even in the worst times she was soft-spoken and calm, and clearly loved her son. At no point did she pass judgment on the nature of his illness. Her southern accent charmed me, and I'd miss my morning discussions with her, even though those discussions had centered on Bill's depressing condition. Despite the stress of caring for him and the relief I felt at his passing, I would also miss Bill. The most difficult period for me had come toward the end when he grew contentious and irritable, testing my patience and forcing me to question my clinical competence. But who wouldn't be contentious and irritable in such a situation? Bill had otherwise been a pleasure to know, and his death filled me with immense sadness.

I didn't linger long in Bill's room because I had other patients to see in the hospital that morning, and I'd promised to visit a patient at home before going to my office. Leaving Bill's mother and David to grieve privately, I frantically tried to round on everyone else before 9:00 a.m. I had a painful conversation with Justin, whom I'd admitted recently for pneumonia. In the past I'd treated him for KS and an infection called MAC, from which he'd recovered. Since admission, his condition had worsened. In addition to pneumonia, his bone marrow was failing—his red and white blood cells and platelets were low, which put him at risk for other serious infections, heart failure, and a life-threatening hemorrhage.

The day after admission I had been compelled to place him in respiratory isolation because a sputum sample showed "red snappers," tuberculosis bacteria, which stain red when tested. Although he probably had a recurrence of MAC, an organism in the same family as tuberculosis but not communicable and, in people with normal immune systems, usually harmless, we presumed old-fashioned TB until proven otherwise. To protect ourselves, we wore tight-fitting masks with pores small enough to prevent penetration by infectious spores. Not only are such masks tight, but they are also malodorous from the smell of one's own trapped breath. Talking through one of these masks is like talking through a tube, which makes one's voice sound hollow and muffled.

Now I had to give Justin bad news through that hot, tight mask: He didn't have tuberculosis. MAC had returned, indicating that his previous treatments for it had failed and that he was likely to die from his infection. I didn't tell him that he'd die from it; I didn't have to, because he knew what the failure of treatment meant. As I spoke, he stared at me in horror and disbelief. Not wanting to hear what I had to say, he fidgeted, coughed, groaned, and backed away from me as if I'd lunged at him with a knife; but he was in bed and had nowhere to go. I tried to grab one of his hands as he folded himself into a ball by the headboard and sobbed. Without that physical connection, no words could console him: I couldn't look him directly in the eye as I spoke, and everything I said seemed pointless. He was too overwhelmed with grief and fear to hear me anyway.

Tall and skinny with peachy skin, a ponytail, a scruffy goatee, and blue eyes, Justin at first had put me off, reminding me of a hippie from the 1960s. In my mind hippies were difficult to deal with because they rejected the status quo and preferred alternatives to everything, including modern medicine. Although to a certain extent that was true for Justin, we'd developed a good rapport. Like

Bill, he was at heart a gentle soul, and I overlooked what I viewed as his eccentricities. But when a doctor has to deliver bad news, a wall drops down and a friend can become an enemy. I felt like a spy whose identity had been exposed, an agent of the AIDS virus, a messenger of death. At the height of the AIDS crisis I'd been typecast in the role of a grim reaper gripping a stethoscope instead of a scythe. Perhaps an actor would have relished the part, but I hated it.

As I tried to speak, Justin hyperventilated and grasped at his oxygen mask as if it were a lifeline. An outpouring of heat from the vents (the building's heating system dated back to the 1960s) had turned the room into a sauna, and sweat poured from his brow and stained his gown. I was sweating too. He squirmed at every word, and I wanted to flee. I felt awkward, as I'd erred in my approach to him. I'd come to his room to discuss end-of-life issues, but end-of-life issues were the last thing he wanted to talk about. Having just dealt with Bill's death, I lacked the energy to press further.

Since there was nothing more for me to say and no way to console him, I left in frustration and sadness, mentally throwing up my hands at the hopelessness of it all. In the charting area I made uncomfortable telephone calls to one of Justin's friends and his mother. It was time for them to come to Chicago, I advised, before Justin "passed away." I avoided giving them a timeline—no one dies on a predictable schedule—but he couldn't survive much longer, especially since I'd run out of medications to prescribe for him.

That night Gavin and I opened a bottle of wine before dinner to help us unwind, which had become a nearly daily ritual. In the winter we'd sit on the white leather couch and armchair in the living room in front of a crackling fire, curtains drawn and Monty begging us to play with him or, when that didn't work, curling up beside us as we talked. In the summer we headed to the second-floor deck that overlooked a shade garden packed with rhododendrons, holly, and hostas and bounded by the garage, whose ivy-carpeted wall seemed to ripple in the breeze. Surrounding us were the back porches of other homes and apartments and the black ropes of telephone and electrical wires, an uninspiring urban landscape. We discussed our work, competing for the worst case or worst experience of the day. Gavin had his share of AIDS cases, but AIDS wasn't the only disease that destroyed the lives of our patients. No one ever won these depressing contests. And alcohol did little to improve our moods. Our preferred addiction was travel, and we often longed to be anywhere but in Chicago. But like any addiction, that form of escape never fully satisfied.

In truth I could never escape, because my mind traveled with me, and in that mind were images of the dead and dying I struggled to suppress or forget. In my darkest moments, my body felt like a prison. Like the boy wounded by a gunshot who had slunk along the fence that one autumn day, I longed to be whisked off to a place of safety, free of stress and anxiety. But for me that place didn't exist.

: 11 :

AIDS in Namibia

(1992–93)

I n the fall of 1992 I decided to examine HIV in a foreign country, a project that would combine my work treating AIDS patients and my passion for international travel. Only a year earlier, in Botswana, I'd dismissed such a project, preferring to be a tourist rather than a physician engaged in clinical research. But now I wanted to look beyond my narrow world.

Despite the horrors that often engulfed me, I found AIDS strangely fascinating. AIDS had replaced syphilis as the so-called Great Imitator. With its potential to affect every organ in the body, just like syphilis, it mimicked other medical problems like heart failure, leukemia, stroke, Alzheimer's disease, or multiple sclerosis. No two patients with the disease were alike, which made HIV both intellectually stimulating and emotionally challenging. When the enthusiasm of my interns and residents flagged under the burden of so many sick young men, I reminded them our work permitted them to learn about the management of all sorts of common health problems, which they could apply to their own patients after completing their training. In those settings the only difference was that HIV wouldn't be the underlying cause of, say, kidney failure, for example. In both scenarios the patient needed dialysis. It was a hard sell.

The impetus for this shift in my focus was a master's program in public health that I enrolled in at the University of Illinois at Chicago. That was in September 1992, at the height of the AIDS crisis, a crazy idea. I already worked fifty to sixty hours per week, not counting calls at night or weekend hospital rounds, but I yearned for a more substantive diversion than a two-week holiday. The addition of C. to our practice in 1991 gave me greater flexibility in scheduling my patients and two weekends off a month. Somehow, I thought, I'd find time to squeeze in classes, take exams, and write papers, while caring for patients and maintaining an active social life.

Public health had interested me since medical school. Some of the greatest advances in medicine had occurred not in the laboratory or operating room but on a larger stage. Edward Jenner's smallpox vaccine and Jonas Salk's polio vaccine eventually halted two of humanity's most devastating epidemics; John Snow, the father of modern epidemiology, the study of the impact of diseases on human populations, traced the source of a cholera outbreak in London to a contaminated water pump and pointed the way toward the establishment of a clean and safe water supply. And the introduction of oral rehydration therapy markedly reduced death rates from diarrhea in infants and children in resource-poor countries. In tandem with advances in medicine—the invention of anesthesia, the elaboration of the germ theory as the basis for infectious diseases, and the discovery of penicillin, to name a few—public health measures had improved the quality of human life and doubled life expectancy in resource-rich countries like the US, Europe, Japan, Australia, and New Zealand from forty years at the turn of the nineteenth century to eighty at the end of the twentieth. AIDS threatened to upend that hard-earned progress.

It might seem odd that I sought to alleviate my stress by returning to the classroom, but I've always been a nerd. I can spend hours roaming through bookstores and libraries, skimming works of fiction and nonfiction that pique my interest, entranced by prose and images that transport me to a different world. Books and intellectual discourse, even on subjects related to my daily work, would be the perfect antidote for my stratospheric stress levels, I hoped, since psychotherapy hadn't done much good and vacations provided only a temporary remedy.

Hearing the news, one of my AIDS patients burst into tears because he thought I was leaving Chicago to work for the World Health Organization in Geneva. I wondered how this rumor got started. Before the advent of social media, gossip spread around the Chicago gay community in the old-fashioned way, by word of mouth. I suppose it was a logical assumption because many of my patients were aware of my penchant for travel. To this patient, a thirty-five-year-old man from Finland, it wasn't farfetched for someone to uproot himself and relocate to a strange land several thousand miles from his birthplace. My grandparents had done that, in what is now Ukraine, escaping with their families from murderous Cossack bands that hunted them like animals because they were Jews. Many gay men from other parts of the world had made a similar exodus, immigrating to the United States because it offered the hope of acceptance and freedom from persecution. Touched by this unexpected outpouring of emotion, I hugged my patient and told him what I was really doing.

But I couldn't promise him I would still be practicing in a few years. I had an additional reason for getting another degree: job security, a funny thing for a doctor to worry about. The fee-for-service model of medical care was coming to an end, because it encouraged too much unnecessary testing or too many procedures, rewarding quantity rather than quality. Up until the early 1980s, hospitals and doctors experienced little regulation. A patient suffering a heart attack might spend weeks on a coronary care unit, and the government (in the case of Medicare) or private insurers footed the bill. Moreover, rapid advances in technology had pushed healthcare costs upward. The costs far outpaced inflation. Something had to be done, and doctors and hospitals were perceived as part of the problem, not the solution. The potential changes sent doctors, including me, who were not used to having their judgment questioned, into a tizzy. Denial of payment for a service or permission to order an MRI, both deemed unnecessary by an unseen reviewer; prior authorization requests for an expensive medication; piles of paperwork; long waiting times to appeal the denials until you just gave up—these were some of the frustrations we were subjected to. I imagined two curves, revenue and expenses, converging over time and eroding my personal income. I hoped the extra credential of an MPH would give me more job options in a changing medical world. Perhaps I could work for the WHO, if I got sick of it all or was driven out of private medical practice.

In the classroom I enjoyed interacting with healthy men and women whose experiences and aspirations differed from my own. It was, metaphorically, like going to a spa in the mountains, if one ignored the Brutalist architecture. Students came from all over the world to attend this program. One young man I developed a bit of a crush on had spent time in Mali on a project to eradicate the guinea worm, a grotesque scourge in West Africa. (A year or more after a person drinks water contaminated by a flea that carries guinea worm larvae, hideous adult worms emerge from blisters on their limbs, causing intense burning pain and sometimes death.) Everyone I met was eager to use what they learned in the program to improve public health in their respective states or countries. I was surprised that the competitive spirit I'd known in college returned in full force. I wouldn't settle for anything less than an A, although it made little difference what grades I got.

Studying the AIDS epidemic as a public health problem, not just a medical condition, became one of my prime objectives during the next two years. At every opportunity I wrote a paper on some aspect of the crisis—AIDS and the law, AIDS in the workplace, and the global dimensions of the AIDS epidemic, among other topics. The academic spirit energized me and gave new meaning to my work as a doctor.

One day in my International Health class we watched a short film called *Land without Bread*, a 1932 documentary by Luis Buñuel that focused on an economically depressed village in Spain. Neglected by the Catholic Church and the Spanish monarchy, people there suffered from malnutrition, poor sanitation, and diseases like goiter due to lack of iodine in their diets and anemia due to iron deficiency, and they died of snakebites, infected wounds, dehydration and dysentery. With dramatic improvements in public health, these problems vanished in two generations. How I wished that we could have solved the AIDS epidemic with equally effective tools!

Before class that morning I'd rounded on five very sick men: Carl, who'd spent most of the last year in the hospital with one difficult medical problem after another; Adam, with a new case of PCP, who'd given up alcohol and cut down his work hours as bargaining chips in his losing battle; Jordan, who'd survived two bouts of PCP and in the previous few days miraculously returned to life after his kidneys had nearly shut down as a result of a dangerous bacterial infection; Alvin, a former body builder admitted for weight loss and fevers, who'd refused AZT and adamantly opposed any measures to prolong his life; and Lane, a polite and dignified man who was dying from multiple opportunistic infections but still retained a sense of humor, replying with a weak smile when asked how he felt, "Like two eggs and a slice of ham."

Although these patients were well cared for, 11 West was in disarray. I did my best to avoid being swept into the drama, but that was impossible. Rod, the head nurse for the last four years and a former priest with whom I helped set up a free-standing facility for homeless AIDS patients called Bonaventure House, had quit and run away to California with a man twenty years younger. The nurse who replaced him, a lesbian, was fired because she was stealing narcotics to help cope with a recent breakup with a girlfriend. We also fired a nurse's aide for arriving to work drunk. Another nurse was suspended for two days without pay because she drove home a known drug abuser who left against medical advice to meet his supplier. Her excuse was that she didn't want him to get hurt, but that didn't sit well. If she'd gotten into an accident with the patient, her supervisor pointed out, the hospital could have been sued. Sometimes AIDS attracted a motley assortment of caregivers who often demanded more attention and tender loving care than the patients they served. But others were rocks. Carol, a wonderful nurse who'd cared for our patients since the beginning of the epidemic and hung on despite the stress, once remarked to one of her dysfunctional fellow caregivers, whose departure seemed imminent, "I was here before you got here and I'll be here long after you're gone."

I admit that my own life during that time was also out of control. *I'm trying to do too much—work, school, social gatherings, opera,* I wrote in my journal in February 1993. *I'm sleeping barely 5 hours a night, and the sleep has been fitful. Too much on my mind. Last Saturday I awoke early to do some homework; I had class 9:30-12: 30; I rushed to the office to see ten patients, until 4 o'clock. We had guests for dinner. Gavin went out to a benefit/party and didn't come home until 3. I had 6 hours to relax on Sunday, then we had a political dinner to go to. . . . On Monday I got to the hospital at 6:30 AM. I had nine patients to see; from 9-10 I attended AIDS rounds. My office schedule was packed. I had umpteen messages. I had class 5-7. I met Tom and C. for dinner at 8, went to sleep at 11, awoke at 5, made rounds, attended class at U of I, rushed back to the office foolishly by way of the expressway, which was bumper to bumper because of construction (I cursed, mumbled to myself, pounded the steering wheel, gnashed my teeth—wondered if anybody could see me and, if they could, wondered if they thought I was nuts), saw patients 1-6:30, picked up Gavin at home to go to the opera, saw a fabulous production of* Das Rheingold *(the Rhine maidens suspended by bungee cords, swimming, dancing in midair), went to sleep at 11, awoke at 5, rounds 6:30-9:00, office 9:00-11:00, drove down to U of I to meet with the instructor of my International Health class who had some slides and literature for me on schistosomiasis [a parasitic disease] for a presentation I offered to make at the end of March . . . ran an errand, got my hair cut, returned to U of I for class, returned home, walked Monty and Fiona, played with them, puttered around till 8:30, met Gavin and two residents for dinner, went to bed at midnight, awoke at 5, dashed off to the hospital at 6:30 . . . and then I began to unravel.*

And yet I didn't unravel. I kept going and pushing on even when my body clamored for rest. I'm not a quitter. "Winners never quit; quitters never win" was a high school gym aphorism that had stuck with me, despite my total lack of athletic ability. It popped into my mind whenever I felt like running away from an unpleasant task or project.

The project I now decided to undertake was an exploration of the impact of the AIDS epidemic on Namibia, in part because of its obscurity to Western audiences. Few of my friends had heard of Namibia, a country half the size of Alaska with a population of just 1.5 million people, and no one I knew had been there. Moreover, little was known about the course of AIDS there. I planned to spend ten days in Namibia in late May 1993, then head to Berlin for the Ninth International Conference on AIDS to learn more about AIDS in southern Africa. There was nothing more for me to learn about AIDS in the West. I'd already filled a file cabinet with alphabetized folders full of articles from numerous journals related to every aspect of AIDS. I felt like a field biologist assembling a menagerie of moths, butterflies, and other insects before the advent of evolutionary theory. *What does it all mean?* I sometimes wondered.

In 1993 Google didn't exist, nor did Amazon.com. Research could be cumbersome: I had to comb libraries for relevant publications and search bookstore catalogs for books about Namibia. There wasn't much. And for reasons that were never made clear to me by the heads of public health clinics or hospital directors I solicited, I would not be allowed to examine patients or visit clinics in Namibia, which would have added a human dimension to my research. That disappointed me because I was a doctor, not a journalist, spy or politician.

Early on I realized that I would have to infer the nature of the epidemic there from statistics gathered in countries that encircled Namibia—Angola, Zambia, Zimbabwe, Botswana, and South Africa, where the epidemic raged. An observer in South Africa prophesied that there "AIDS will knock the bottom out of health budgets." Already many hospital beds in other sub-Saharan countries were occupied by patients with HIV-related problems. For example, at the University Teaching Hospital in Lusaka, Zambia, people with AIDS occupied 40–60 percent of the beds, not much different from American cities with sizable gay populations. In Botswana, just under half of hospitalized patients with tuberculosis were HIV positive. There was no reason for me to expect the situation to be different in Namibia.

Namibia had become a sovereign nation only three years earlier, in March 1990, after seventy years of racially separatist South African domination. Before that it had been a German colony for thirty years. A small urban white population still spoke German as their primary language. Since independence, Namibia had become a multiparty democracy.

Overall, Namibia is arid. The parched landscape, rugged topography, and quality of light surrounding its capital, Windhoek, reminded me of northern New Mexico. The sky was cloudless and the air pollution-free. Scrubby plants sprouted from the sandy, iron-stained soil. The most distinctive geological features were inselbergs, which resembled islands of weathered crags. At sunset the earth turned a kaleidoscope of colors from the fine dust in the atmosphere. It looked like nothing could flourish here, not even AIDS.

Yet Windhoek was picturesque in a way that seemed more European than African. It did not conjure up the American perceptions of Africa as poor, dependent, and even barbaric. Rather, it brimmed with busy shops, and well-dressed people both white and black crowded the streets. The tidiness and prosperity of Windhoek impressed me, until I learned that 70 percent of Namibia's people lived in impoverished rural areas and 75 percent of the wealth was controlled by only 5 percent of the people. Trying to expand its tourism industry, Namibia had opened itself to Western journalists. Only a week before leaving Chicago, I read two articles about Namibia in the *New York Times*, one about the disappearance of the San culture (Bushmen) in the Caprivi Strip, a panhandle stretching northeast to Zimbabwe; another about an American couple who'd moved to Namibia to save the dwindling cheetah population.

But to my chagrin, Namibia was a homophobic country. When Gavin and I arrived at our hotel, the clerk ignored our request for a single room and consigned us to separate but adjacent rooms. We slept in one bed anyway, locking the door to prevent accidental entry of a maid. We messed up the bed in the other room and bathroom, strategically placing pubic hairs in both to give the illusion that we slept and bathed separately. During our travels there our guide, a white Namibian, made sure that Gavin and I didn't share a tent. When one of our fellow travelers, an eccentric elderly American woman Peace Corps volunteer, remarked to our guide—who helped set up camp, cook our food, and ensure our comfort—that he would make a good "househusband," he replied with a limp wrist. Another white Namibian in the group added, "We don't have any of those here. They're all in San Francisco." Although it wasn't necessarily dangerous to be a gay traveler in Namibia, gays weren't welcome—though this could be true in the United States too. Acceptance and tolerance were relative concepts, codified in constitutions that guaranteed equal rights for all citizens but ignored in practice.

My first research task was to meet with Dr. Markus Goraseb, the AIDS Programme director. I knew nothing about his background or who employed him. I'd drawn up a list of forty questions to help me understand the recent social and political changes that had contributed to the spread of the AIDS virus there. I was searching for solid statistics. In light of the lack of discussion in the medical literature, I had little choice but to rely on my Namibian sources if I was to learn anything substantive. But prior to my arrival they hadn't been forthcoming. A fax to the AIDS Programme the week before had gone unanswered. My only lead had come from the World Bank, where my contact sent me publications about health problems and economic indicators of Namibia, although she cautioned me not to mention the statistics to anyone since they had not yet been released to the Namibian government. She also recommended that I visit the UNICEF office in Windhoek, which was likely to have statistics on a variety of health factors. It was she who had given me Dr. Goraseb's name.

From my hotel, I hailed a cab but had no idea where I was going. The taxi driver dropped me off somewhere and pointed me toward the Christ Lutheran Church, a local landmark, by the Parliament building. I walked up a slight incline but then didn't know where to go. I found my way to the Ministry of Agriculture, where a thin, affable older black man stood by the entrance. I asked him for directions to the public hospital.

"Oh no, no, sir. It's very far away, all the way across town," he said in accented English. My heart sank. He said it was too far to walk, but I wasn't sure I believed him. I asked for a telephone and he led me inside, to the minister's office. A pleasant white secretary confirmed the man's directions, which made me feel sheepish for distrusting him. Thanking them both, I found another taxi. The driver needed more gas, which made me nervous because already I was at risk of arriving late for my appointment, but nevertheless we soon arrived at a rambling, austere series of low-lying buildings.

It took three different people to direct me to Dr. Goraseb's office. I could tell I was close because there were posters on the wall addressing the AIDS problem. Then, to my chagrin, no one knew where Dr. Goraseb was or when he was due to arrive. I wondered if I'd wasted my time. In the interim, a secretary directed me to a Dr. Boadu, a short, stocky man dressed informally in a short-sleeved shirt. Caught off guard, he asked for my credentials before promising to talk to me in five minutes. He led me to a conference room adjacent to his office where I could wait for him. That room looked out onto a tidy courtyard landscaped with various shrubs and flowers. On a large pad of paper on an easel, someone had scribbled something like "AIDS is Yth," a picture of a face, and the word "ignorance." I wasn't sure what it meant, but it presumably addressed the fact that the ignorance of young people drove the epidemic in Namibia. There were also a few posters, among them an advertisement for World Health Day and a cartoon of a man and woman discussing safe sex. I discovered a library of sorts, a set of pigeonholes with pamphlets on AIDS and HIV. Some pamphlets originated from the CDC, WHO, or other governmental sources in Africa, all outlining policies or recommending policies or approaches to the AIDS problem.

I waited about thirty minutes. I could hear Dr. Boadu speaking to various people. Eventually he entered with a middle-aged female secretary and a handsome young black man sporting rimless spectacles who introduced himself as Tsali. Currently a student at Denison University in Ohio who hoped to go to medical school, Tsali had an interest in epidemiology and was researching health problems in Namibia. He'd only been in Namibia for a few weeks. It had been six years since his last visit to his homeland.

Speaking at a rapid clip, Dr. Boadu gave us a history of the AIDS problem in Namibia, repeating what I'd gleaned from the pamphlets. Thus far 4,400 cases had been reported, but he emphasized that these "stats" were meaningless. Who knew how many? he said. Diagnoses were made using the WHO-Bangui definition of AIDS: weight loss greater than 10 percent of baseline body weight; chronic diarrhea for more than a month; prolonged fever for more than a month; and other physical signs of immune suppression in the absence of another known cause. He couldn't tell me what major indicator diseases in Namibia were, because AIDS was still a "clinical" diagnosis—based on signs and symptoms rather than on laboratory tests, which were often too expensive to run.

He talked about Namibia's plans and goals, which remained notional because funds were short, though various nongovernmental organizations and government agencies had pledged financial support. Because of limitations in access and cost, HIV testing was not widespread, he said, but it was done for prenatal care. However, since many people didn't go to hospitals for their medical care, he had little hard data.

Dr. Boadu didn't seem to harbor the common prejudice in Africa about the homosexual transmission of HIV in the West, nor did he dismiss the role of traditional healers in Namibian health care. He himself was Ghanaian, a fact that implied that Namibia lacked the medical personnel or expertise to confront the epidemic, which might have explained why I wasn't allowed to see patients. Because he was in a great hurry, I never saw his credentials. He left us in the hands of the secretary, who knew a good deal more about HIV/AIDS than I expected. She happily agreed to make copies of some documents for me.

Tsali drove me back to the center of town. He told me that he had two brothers, one also in the United States studying law, the other a ten-year-old who was at home with their parents. His family had befriended the American couple helping to save the cheetah. Although he didn't acknowledge it, his family belonged to the ruling elite. His father held an important job, the nature of which was not revealed to me.

Tsali was very bright and clear-headed. He was determined to become a doctor and return to help his country. He told me that he intended to remain in Africa until August before returning to the US. I promised to send him some articles about health problems in Namibia, but I hesitated to extend an invitation to Chicago because I didn't know his attitude toward gay people. Perhaps he was also gay. It was hard to tell. Sometimes in foreign countries I thought all the men were gay. They were far more affectionate with their friends, wore better clothes and hipper hairstyles, and rarely walked with a swagger like young men did in the United States. But American gay men emulated Europeans in style and manner, not vice versa.

Back at the hotel, I collected Gavin and we mistakenly hunted for the UNICEF office in the Ministry of Justice. We wandered down a short, dim hallway lined with posters, mainly of wildlife. A man at a desk called out to us, his voice echoing. He had no idea about UNICEF, but he was kind enough to find out and give us directions. As we left, we noticed an anti-AIDS poster sponsored by an Islamic group, which blasted the West for telling people to have fun and be gay and to have lots of sex. It also condemned condoms and advocated abstinence. Gavin and I snickered at its clumsy cartoons. The posters would have had negligible effect in Namibia itself, because less than 1 percent of the population there was Muslim.

At UNICEF headquarters a clerk handed us blue badges, which we each clipped onto a lapel. Gavin waited in the lobby while a friendly secretary led me to the office of the medical director. Although I'd made an appointment weeks in advance and traveled thousands of miles to meet with him, he, like Dr. Goraseb, wasn't available. Sensing my disappointment, his secretary allowed me to peruse various documents in a little library. Delighted to find so many relevant publications, I quickly forgot the slight. With permission, I started copying one of the documents but quickly realized I'd never finish, given my time constraints. I was able to cajole a young woman working in the library to make copies of three of them, each less than twenty-five pages long. Then we sat and talked about my project, which interested her.

She spoke about the difficulties of educating Namibians about AIDS. AIDS was a disease of young people, she said. When it came to sex, there was no parental guidance. The men, like men all over the world, gay or straight, didn't want to wear condoms. Well educated and fairly sophisticated, she seemed to enjoy chatting about her country, even about such morbid subjects as AIDS. In fact, after a while I wondered if I'd be able to leave. Finally I managed to thank her for her help and kindness, return to the lobby, and drag Gavin, whose patience had been stretched to a tether, to another bookstore in search of a book she had recommended.

We spent the next five days traveling throughout the country by air and Land Rover, encountering herds of elephants, various antelopes, zebras, and giraffe but no lions or big cats. For the most part we had the highway to ourselves. When a vehicle sped by, it was most often a Mercedes Benz, BMW, or Audi with white driver and occupants. Now and then a truck roared past heading for I knew not where, the driver invariably black. I wondered if the trucks left Namibia for Botswana, Zambia, or places even farther afield. I needed to find out, because in Africa AIDS spread along truck routes. Trucks there were the modern equivalents of caravans traversing the Silk Road and flotillas invading Asia and the Americas, conveying material goods, religion, and disease from one part of the globe to another.

Near a town called Otavi we stopped at a rundown roadside filling station. I glimpsed a few black men loitering outside the toilets. A black woman in a skimpy dress with shoulder straps and a low neckline teased them. It was clear that she was a prostitute and the filling station an informal truck stop. Here was a vivid example of how an epidemic spreads. An apparently healthy woman (or man) and apparently clear water differ little when it comes to disease transmission. People drink at both wells without hesitation. If a virus or bacterium loomed as large as monsters, who wouldn't flee? But viruses and bacteria are invisible to the naked eye. It takes imagination, experience, and a belief in the discoveries of modern science to fear infectious agents, which we can't see. To many people in the world the idea of a human being as a vector of a lethal disease seems incomprehensible. It's as if a gas chamber at Auschwitz masqueraded as a cleansing shower for the unsuspecting victims who were directed there to clean up immediately after their arrival.

Back in Windhoek, we parked our van on a major thoroughfare. We'd been cautioned about the prevalence of theft in the city, and the barbed wire and broken bottles atop the walled enclaves along our trip attested to a high rate of burglaries. If potential thieves peered through the darkened windows of our vehicle, they could see our luggage, which included books, pamphlets, and other important research documents. I didn't care about the clothes or toiletries, which could be replaced, but the books and papers were irreplaceable. Gavin told me to stop worrying. We dined at a café on the second floor of a building from which we could see the van. Although Gavin thought I was being paranoid, he promised not to let the van out of his sight.

The café bustled with activity. Most of the customers were tourists or expats, and we caught bits of their conversation. A group of American women detailed their sexual exploits in San Diego. *Thank God they weren't gay men*, I thought, *or they might have freaked out about their health instead.* By coincidence, the man who'd organized one of our tours dined nearby with his wife. As we thanked him for a wonderful trip, Gavin's attention suddenly returned to the van, which two suspicious-looking men were scoping out. Without excusing himself, he dashed out of the restaurant, while I continued to chat with the couple and tried not to appear nervous. After shaking their hands, I paid our bill and left in a rush.

The street teemed with people and was blocked off because of some sort of charity parade that the country's president planned to attend. I seemed to be the only person moving in the direction of our car. By the time I reached the car, after what seemed to be an eternity because of my anxiety, Gavin fumed in the driver's seat, gripping the steering wheel. The two men had been looking to break in, but when he shooed them, they wouldn't leave until he became enraged. He admitted to being unnerved because they could have been armed with guns or knives, though violent crime in Windhoek was rare.

The incident hardly marred the trip. As we drove to the distant airport to catch our flight to Berlin, we traveled a lonely highway that followed the contours of the scrubby rolling hills and talked about what it might be like to live in Namibia working for some nongovernmental medical organization. We wouldn't have brought anything valuable, we agreed. Although Windhoek was still quaint, belying the quaintness were the poverty and misery of the majority of the population. In those impoverished townships, with their rudimentary healthcare services and widespread ignorance about safe sex practices, an epidemic like AIDS would be unstoppable.

: 12 :

AIDS in Berlin

(1993)

We arrived in Berlin on a Sunday morning in the first week of June 1993. Most of the people flying in then were heading to the AIDS conference. It was a truly international array of visitors from the Americas, Asia, Africa, and other parts of Europe. I admit that I wasn't excited about being in Berlin, though Gavin was. Because of Hitler and the Holocaust, Germany ranked near the bottom of places I wanted to explore. I had come to attend the conference, not to immerse myself in the country's history and culture or mingle with its inhabitants.

This was my fourth international AIDS conference, after Paris in 1986, San Francisco in 1990, and Florence in 1991. Although conferences had been held in the United States, no future ones were planned there because of its restrictive and regressive immigration policies: HIV-positive individuals from foreign countries were forbidden to enter. This outraged the sponsors of the annual event, the International AIDS Society and the World Health Organization. I was outraged too, but I wasn't an activist. I didn't fire off letters in protest or march with ACT-UP. Instead I grumbled about its outrageousness to patients and colleagues, like an armchair politician. President Barack Obama finally rescinded that policy in 2010.

Our hotel was in the former East Berlin, which had been liberated from the Soviet sphere only four years earlier. After showering and changing, we set out for the International Conference Center in West Berlin to register for the week's events. As we left the hotel, we paused to admire a grand building with a frieze on its architrave and a blackened dome adorned with bronze emblems that gleamed in the sunlight. The rest of the neighborhood was in the throes of gentrification, its streets shredded to make way for modern sewers and buildings cocooned in various stages of restoration. In five to ten years the entire area would be unrecognizable, the grime replaced with glitz. Already fancy boutiques had moved in. There was even a Mercedes-Benz dealership. As we took the elevated train, the amount of graffiti I could see appalled me. Gibberish and hideous slashes of paint covered every available surface and spared no building. I wondered why the municipal government and Berlin's citizens tolerated such brazen defacement of public and private property. Its ubiquity disturbed me, as if chaos were triumphing over order. Like most doctors, I prefer order.

The ICC was an ugly futuristic building constructed of steel and glass. Security guards, anticipating outbursts from AIDS activists, were everywhere and made the place more forbidding. The wan light of fluorescent bulbs illuminated the halls and rooms, as in any modern convention center. Navigation would be tricky, I thought. The interior was multitiered with stairs and escalators radiating in every direction. Thousands of people would be attending, adding to the disorder. Already they milled around everywhere, carrying black shoulder bags emblazoned with the orange logo of the conference, Halloween colors in late spring.

The conference itself, which began the next morning, depressed me. It had no particular theme and at times seemed more like a carnival than a solemn gathering of sincere individuals united to combat a deadly disease. I struggled to drum up excitement as each sad day passed. In the opening lecture Dr. Michael Merson, the director of WHO's Global Programme on AIDS, set a pessimistic tone by declaring that millions of people worldwide had been infected with HIV despite all the efforts of to control its spread. In all ways, he said, the pandemic was truly global in scope. Although we'd learned much about how to help people avoid behavior that put them at risk of sexual and blood-borne transmission of HIV, such measures alone were insufficient to slow the pace of new infections. Political leaders had vastly underfunded efforts to find effective treatments and curb risky behavior. Without greater commitment AIDS could not be controlled, he warned. In another lecture Dr. J. M. A. Lange from Holland offered a glimmer of hope that there were promising new drugs and drug combinations on the horizon. But the effects of monotherapy—that is, the use of a single agent like AZT to treat HIV—were modest and transient, Dr. I. V. D. Weller concluded. It's not surprising that I found myself much more interested in global public health issues than basic or even clinical sciences.

Every day saw a breakfast meeting sponsored by Burroughs Wellcome, the pharmaceutical giant that marketed AZT. These were intended to bring more than one hundred clinicians and experts together to review the previous day's presentations with the goal of producing a booklet for American physicians caring for people with HIV/AIDS. There was a time in the earliest years of the epidemic when I was honored to participate in these affairs and hobnob with the AIDS glitterati, the movers and shakers in the scientific community from San Francisco, Los Angeles, New York, and Chicago who'd been the first responders in the war against AIDS. Because of the number of AIDS patients in my practice, I was feted like an important person, first by infectious disease specialists in Chicago who needed patients for their scientific studies, then by companies that developed treatments for opportunistic infections, and now by companies that marketed treatments against the virus itself. Pharmaceutical reps courted and flattered me, invited me to dinners at expensive restaurants, and paid me a stipend for conducting community forums at which I would speak about AIDS to audiences of vulnerable gay men. I sat on so-called advisory boards with colleagues from around the country, expressing my opinion about the value of a particular medication or the direction research should take. I enjoyed the limelight yet felt a bit like one of the Beverly Hillbillies, fawned over because of their accidental wealth.

But by 1993 I was no longer enamored. A few of the glitterati had morphed into nothing more than Burroughs Wellcome whores, I thought, paid hefty sums for their time and effort. Unfortunately, Big Pharma influenced them too profoundly. A pioneering AIDS physician from one of the university hospitals in California headed my breakfast table. For a member of the glitterati he was a very pleasant man, down-to-earth, personable, and genuinely concerned about the welfare of his patients. Sometimes one had to make a pact with the devil to advance a scientific cause, I mused. The other physicians at my table, mostly infectious disease specialists, were also amiable. I was the only primary care physician, the lowest man on the totem pole, a foot soldier, not a high-ranking officer, in the war against AIDS. At times I was just a hot mess, full of contradictions and inconsistencies. One moment I hated being in the limelight because my ego wasn't large enough to embrace and enjoy it. The next moment that same ego bristled at the thought that the glitterati and other infectious disease specialists didn't take me seriously as an expert on equal footing with them.

The results of the Concorde Study dominated the conference. Essentially, the study demonstrated that AZT alone in patients who had no symptoms of HIV did not improve survival or impede progression to AIDS. Following the CD4 count (known less accurately but more commonly as the T cell count) was not a useful marker for success of therapy, though the count tended to rise in those who took the medication, hinting at a beneficial effect on the immune system. Dr. Maxime Seligmann, a respected French immunologist, presented a detailed analysis of the study, taking care not to extrapolate the findings to individuals with symptoms of HIV or to the possible effectiveness of drug combinations. But other data about combinations of anti-HIV agents were equally disappointing, he said.

What was I to tell my patients when I returned to my practice? What hope could I offer them? Did I continue to cling to AZT despite the Concorde study, and despite the fact that AZT was expensive and some insurance companies refused to cover it? When it was not covered, only the wealthiest people could afford AZT, though now it seemed that they'd squandered their money anyway.

We discussed little else at the breakfast sessions. By the end of the conference many of us felt frustrated, confused, and defeated. Despite the negative data, some of the glitterati stuck by AZT, insisting on its efficacy. *How difficult it is to give up something you've spent years supporting!* I thought. *I should know something about that psychological phenomenon. How much time did I waste trying to salvage my relationship with Art despite the odds against its success? Too long!* With the deepest sincerity, we had all wanted to believe that AZT could save our patients. AZT was released as an investigational drug in 1986; ddI and ddC, similar drugs, followed a few years later. The results of the Concorde study confirmed what most of my colleagues and I now believed: these three medications were ineffective in stopping the progression of AIDS. Yet I had to prescribe something for my patients.

There were interesting, if less sensational, presentations on the pathogenesis (the causal mechanism) and immunology of HIV infection by Dr. Anthony Fauci, from the National Institute of Allergy and Infectious Diseases at the National Institutes of Health, and Dr. Jay Levy, from the University of California at San Francisco. I couldn't say that I understood them thoroughly, but I left impressed with the breadth of our collective knowledge and the progress in understanding the natural history of HIV/AIDS. Dr. Robert Gallo and Dr. Luc Montagnier, who'd carried on a dispiriting battle about priority in the discovery of HIV as the cause of AIDS, also made presentations. Dr. Gallo came across as a cowboy with his antics on stage — the loud voice, the exaggerated expressions, and a flair for the histrionic. Dr. Montagnier, a less flamboyant figure, was incomprehensible, and not because of his French accent or a poor command of English. I comprehended every word, not the content. Perhaps he described some sort of medical or scientific breakthrough, but I wouldn't have known it.

The short lectures varied in quality. Some were downright terrible because of the disorganization of the presenter, obscure topic for discussion, or meager data. I searched in vain for gems among the stones. And the poster sessions were formidable, five thousand of them, I heard. I could review only a handful of them before I succumbed to sensory overload. "Plasma Fibronectin Levels and

Prophylactic Use of Intravenous Gammaglobulin in Children with HIV-1 Infection"; "Use of Microculture Technique for HIV Isolation from Peripheral Blood Mononuclear Cells (PBMC) of Infected Person"—to name a couple at random. My brain overheated and I felt overwhelmed.

Because of my focus on Namibia, I concentrated on presentations from Africa. I was impressed by the sheer volume of small studies conducted there. How difficult it must have been for these individuals to get to Berlin, and how expensive it must have been for private and public institutions to support them. Because of the size and scope of the conference, I wound up missing a presentation by Dr. Boadu from Namibia, who discussed the role of traditional healers in the transmission of HIV. I would have enjoyed speaking to him afterward.

The activists were ubiquitous. On the first day they rushed the main stage with a banner emblazoned with "Tear down the walls!" Adorning themselves with accoutrements of the marginalized—earrings, punk hairstyles, leather bands around their wrists and ankles—they chanted and shouted slogans until security officers dragged them away. I didn't know who these people were or where they came from. They weren't people I interacted with. I had a hard time taking them seriously at first; they seemed too farcical.

But the activists raised valid points. A flyer that members of ACT-UP, AIDS ACTION BALTIMORE, and TAG (Treatment Action Group) distributed targeted a pharmaceutical company, Hoffman LaRoche (HLR), that marketed one drug (ddC), had two others in the pipeline, and had developed a novel test (PCR) to measure the amount of HIV in an infected patient's blood. Although HLR had brought ddC to market in record time after FDA approval, it had made no firm commitment for a larger trial to establish ddC's effectiveness against HIV. Two years after conducting trials on another promising HIV medication, HLR still had released no data.

"Why the stall tactics?" the activists asked, accusing HLR of using US government funds to support its research while stockholders benefited from the enormous profit it derived from its potential medications and diagnostic tools, and then proclaimed,

"THE WORLD WILL NOT PERMIT ROBBER BARON DRUG COMPANIES LIKE HLR TO MAKE HUGE PROFITS AT THE EXPENSE OF PEOPLE WITH HIV AND AIDS. HLR MUST STOP DEVELOPING ITS PROMISING AIDS COMPOUNDS ON-THE-CHEAP!"

Ironically, earlier rebels like Martin Delaney from Project Inform in San Francisco now seemed mainstream. A knowledgeable and articulate nonphysician, Delaney shared the podium with leading immunologists, infectious disease experts, and epidemiologists to discuss the value and limitations of community-based research. That conversation was directed toward groups like the one I belonged to, CPCRA (Community Programs for Clinical Research on AIDS), a consortium of HIV/AIDS practitioners throughout Chicago that I'd help set up. Was our organization, which included similar groups of clinicians from around the country, going to compete with academic and government research centers for scarce dollars or focus on testing unorthodox therapies in common use by HIV-infected gay men and community standards of care, as originally conceived? I agreed with him that we were losing our identity, but the management of AIDS was changing so rapidly that studies we designed became obsolete by the time an oversight committee approved them.

I thought the organizers of the conference were wise to have included the voices of the disenfranchised. But what more could be done to satisfy the protestors? I wondered. Although their level of frustration was understandable, their demands sometimes seemed unreasonable to me.

On the penultimate day of the conference, protestors heckled Dr. F., one of the glitterati from the University of Miami. An enraged HIV-infected physician asked her what he was to do, having wasted two years of his life on ddC and AZT. How could she be so positive about her data, which showed that AZT improved life expectancy as compared to a placebo? When he added, "Your data is invalid because it wasn't analyzed by intent-to-treat" (that is, didn't include people who'd dropped out of the study for one reason or another, which made the data appear better than they were), someone shouted, "Intent-to-cheat, intent-to-cheat!" Dr. F. responded in a tremulous voice, less from intimidation than from anger. "Why direct your anger at me?" she asked. "No one's claiming that these drugs are panaceas!"

HLR wasn't the protestors' only villain. Astra Pharmaceuticals also came under fire for the astronomical cost of Foscavir, a new treatment for CMV retinitis. At one point a hostile crowd surrounded Astra's booth in the conference hall like vengeful bees swarming around someone plundering honey from their hive, forcing the marketing team to flee. Deathly black stickers with a slogan I don't recall were plastered onto the display's tottering walls.

The meeting was such an odd mixture of people: citizens of the resource-rich and resource-poor countries; men and women; gays and straights; world-class scientists and humble clinicians; well-coiffed pharmaceutical representatives and ragamuffin activists. *One world, one humanity*, I thought. AIDS threaded through our social fabric, stitching together the disparate elements into an ungainly giant garment.

Doctors strive to give their patients hope; terminally ill people yearn for a cure; pharmaceutical companies lust for profits. *This combination of cross-purposes has pushed medications onto the market too quickly*, I thought. *Look how much money we've spent on these drugs and yet how little benefit patients derive from them.* In desperation patients would continue to search for alternative, unproven therapies in even greater numbers, I imagined. It was an interesting fact that European AIDS specialists hadn't embraced AZT. We Americans had bought into the Big Pharma model with a vengeance.

In resource-poor countries, people were fatalistic. Every day thousands died of diseases that we in resource-rich countries could treat, like pneumonia or malaria. Thirty percent of the global population had been exposed to tuberculosis, 75 percent of them in the so-called Third World, or resource-poor countries. HIV-infected individuals died of treatable diseases long before they developed untreatable ones. The Concorde study meant nothing to Africans or

Asians, who could barely afford aspirin. To them our debates about it must have seemed ludicrous or gratuitous.

As much as I railed against the sell-out glitterati, I was a bit of a sell-out too. One evening I attended a reception at the Museum of Natural History in East Berlin sponsored by Caremark, a corporation that supplied many of the intravenous solutions and medical equipment for treating my patients at home or in the outpatient setting. We sipped wine and munched on appetizers amid dinosaur skeletons and didn't complain about the ungodly cost of such a frivolous event.

I left Berlin with no new information and little hope for those I cared for. My reflections shifted into a darker sphere. *AIDS mirrored our times*, I penned in my journal. *AIDS seemed like one more marker in humanity's road to destruction. As we reached our carrying capacity on Earth, we were starving ourselves, polluting our environment, threatening to destroy ourselves with nuclear weapons, and now there was a new plague. We couldn't support ourselves on this planet with our current and projected numbers. By the time we fully comprehended these problems as a species, it would be too late. Humans were as destructive as any giant asteroid or massive volcanic eruption [in] the planet's distant past. All species had a carrying capacity. They proliferated until the ecosystem could no longer sustain them, and then the imbalance corrected itself. As a species, we would probably vanish.* Such was my mood that second week of June 1993.

But my experiences in Namibia and Berlin weren't pointless, at least from a personal perspective. With encouragement from my advisor at UIC, I cobbled together my findings in a paper that I published two years later. "As Namibia formulates its national strategy for health care, struggling to guarantee health care and equal access for all, and seeks out funding from shriveling sources for the implementation of its AIDS guidelines," I concluded, "the HIV virus continues its relentless spread into susceptible populations. These strategies will take years to evolve, a period of time the country can ill afford if it hopes to wrest some control over what is rapidly becoming one of the greatest worldwide public health crises of this century."

It was my first and last scientific paper. For me, academia was becoming a dead end. By choice and by necessity, I continued instead down a road with no end in sight.

: 13 :

Turning Point
(1996–2004)

Bruce refused to die. Once athletic and well toned—in his spare time he taught spin classes—by January 1996 he'd become skeletal, like most AIDS patients at the end of their lives. His eye sockets were hollow, his cheeks were sunken, and the skin of his face was drawn tightly like a membrane of a drum stretched over a hollow shell. His sticklike arms and legs protruded from a hospital gown that seemed far too large for his shrunken frame. His situation was beyond hope, yet he couldn't let go; his parents wouldn't let go. They begged me to do everything I could to save his life.

In the 1980s I saw Bruce intermittently for minor ailments. In May 1991 I declared him at the age of thirty-four to be "healthy," although I didn't know his HIV status because he turned down my requests to test him. Without effective treatment at the time, I didn't press the issue. But between that visit and the next one, nearly two years later, he'd been diagnosed with AIDS after hospitalization in the suburbs for PCP. Just before his February 1, 1993, office visit, a test showed profound immune suppression. He could tolerate only half the recommended dose of AZT because he claimed it caused anxiety, but I urged him to increase the dose and added another anti-HIV medication and three others to prevent other opportunistic infections.

During the next two years, Bruce took his medications intermittently and gradually deteriorated, developing dysentery from the cryptosporidium parasite—the same parasite that had contributed to Art's death a decade earlier—and a severe herpes infection in his esophagus. It was difficult for him to swallow without piercing pain, and he could barely drink enough fluids to offset the relentless flow of diarrhea. In December 1995 I admitted him to 11 West because of headaches, problems with balance, and an inability to coordinate the muscles of his eyes. He'd fallen numerous times at home, breaking a glass coffee table on one occasion, and could no longer drive. A brain scan showed lesions that looked suspicious for an untreatable brain infection called PML that killed almost everyone afflicted. Too weak to sit in a wheelchair, he had to be transported from test to test on a gurney. I considered referring him for hospice care.

James, one of 11 West's social workers, met with Bruce and his sister to draw up a power of attorney to determine who would act on his behalf if he could no longer make decisions. They decided that his mother would take responsibility for his health care and his father his condominium. Because of profound weakness in his right arm, Bruce had just enough power to make a few indecipherable cross-hatches. The organism causing PML had damaged the center of his brain that controlled movement in his right arm and leg, like someone who'd had a stroke. It also affected his speech, which was garbled, and I had trouble understanding him. In frustration he mumbled more loudly, which did nothing to make him more comprehensible because he tripped over words and dropped whole syllables or vowels.

In planning for his eventual discharge, Bruce agreed to have a visiting home health aide because he lived alone; no one mentioned hospice to him yet. His mother, who'd just been diagnosed with breast cancer, cried during a private meeting with James and pleaded with him not to let her son know his prognosis. But Bruce was fully aware of his condition and its prognosis. How the two of them would cope in the upcoming months was hard for me to imagine. Nothing I said consoled them. Fortunately, Bruce's sister and father remained level headed throughout the ordeal with their unflagging love and support for Bruce and his mother.

Someone, not I, told Bruce that he had "eight months" to live, and Bruce couldn't get that number out of his head. He was going to beat this thing, he said. I didn't contradict him. Over time I've learned that doctors, myself included, are often wrong about the precise timing of a person's death. There have been times when I thought a person couldn't survive more than a few days, yet after several weeks he was still alive. Or death came in days when it seemed that it would not occur for months. When patients ask me how long they have to live, I parse my words carefully. I'll tell them that eight months, three years, or even ten years is too short for a man or woman in the prime of their life who ordinarily could expect to live to about eighty. In the early days of the AIDS epidemic, such news was more than most people could bear. By the mid-1990s it was less of a shock. Most of my patients with AIDS had already lost a good number of friends to the disease. Although it is hardly a consolation, I assure them that I'll do everything in my power to keep them as comfortable as possible during the process of dying with plenty of narcotics if needed. Such uncertainty distresses people. Once we've reached the acceptance stage of our terminal illness, humans deal better with concrete information, no matter how horrible the news.

After settling matters related to his long-term care, I discharged Bruce to his parents' home. While there he fell down several times and couldn't get up, which he blamed on restarting AZT rather than on his HIV infection. He also lost control of his bladder. His mother requested a bench for the bathtub and a four-pronged cane to help him walk. After reducing his AZT to only one pill a day, instead of the six I'd advised, he wanted to try something else. At the end of January 1996, Bruce's disability was too much for his parents to manage and I readmitted him to 11 West. He was still fully capable of making decisions about his health care, and after a long discussion I convinced him to accept the assistance of Horizon Hospice, but he wanted to go back to his apartment and not to a hospice facility. I delayed discharging him until I could guarantee twenty-four-hour care, wherever he chose to go. I compromised by releasing him back to his parents and having an aide assist him at night, with periodic visits by the hospice nurse.

Before discharge, Bruce asked me about a promising and recently approved anti-HIV drug, Invirase. Invirase belonged to a class of medications called protease inhibitors and seemed most effective when combined with two other anti-HIV agents. Monotherapy—the use of one drug to combat HIV—had proved to be ineffective; dual therapy also seemed ineffective. Scientists hoped that the combination of three medications would be powerful enough to suppress the AIDS virus, a strategy that worked in treating tuberculosis. I doubted that Invirase would help Bruce at this late point in his illness, but I agreed to order it for him.

During a home visit a few days later, the visiting hospice nurse expressed concern that Bruce was in denial about his illness because he insisted that he would get better. I agreed with her assessment. Despite the obvious need for twenty-four-hour care—he was too infirm for his parents to handle alone; they couldn't afford to hire full-time professional caregivers—Bruce refused to leave his parents' house. Although overwhelmed and feeling guilty about her inadequacy as a caregiver, and struggling with her breast cancer, his mother concurred with him. In mid-February when he requested an end to home physical therapy because he could supposedly walk to the bathroom on his own, I noted in his chart, "Whatever he wants. I give up!"

One week later his parents brought Bruce to my office in a wheelchair, his head lolling on his neck like a fruit too heavy for its stalk. He couldn't begin Invirase yet because of a potentially significant interaction with a medication a dermatologist had prescribed to treat pimples on his face, a problem that seemed minor to me in comparison, but Bruce was in charge of his health care, not I. Without doing anything about his HIV infection, he seemed slightly better, though he remained tremulous and couldn't walk without assistance. I promised to order Invirase after he finished the dermatological medication, which he did a week later. He called to remind me to phone the pharmacy. The hospice nurse questioned my order because it was unusual to provide expensive treatments (Invirase cost nearly a thousand dollars per month) for a terminally ill patient. She wondered whether hospice care was still appropriate for him.

In the space of a decade, Horizon Hospice had lost its flexibility in dealing with AIDS patients. In the 1980s a homebound terminally ill young AIDS patient could receive intravenous nutritional support and medications to treat or prevent opportunistic infections with full support from hospice. In that extraordinary setting such treatments and end-of-life care were not viewed as incompatible. But concerns by Medicare and third-party payers about skyrocketing healthcare costs put an end to that practice. Hospices were given a limited budget to care for the dying patient; expenses beyond that had to be covered by the hospice, which threatened to drive them out of business. If hospices cared for people in the terminal phase of their illness, why should they administer expensive therapies that didn't alter the course of the disease? It was a reasonable question to ask. The answer was difficult to deliver, especially to a thirty-year-old man who wasn't ready to die and who rejected the heartlessness of the bottom line.

One month after starting Invirase, Bruce came to see me with a cough. He no longer needed a wheelchair but could walk arm in arm with his parents. His mother, despite her own illness, accompanied Bruce to every visit with me. Although she looked worn from chemotherapy and was beginning to lose her hair, she never complained to me about her health. Bruce didn't always make it easy for her. A few days later a social worker from Horizon described Bruce as "angry and nasty and racist" after he hurled racial epithets at one of the health aides. That was the end of hospice services for Bruce.

Treating Bruce's HIV infection during the next three months was nerve wracking for me. A neurologist at Northwestern whom he consulted for his brain infection recommended higher doses of AZT, to levels that could cause significant side effects, because AZT had been shown to cross into the brain and ameliorate HIV-related neurological symptoms. Calling this good news, Bruce was ready to take AZT again, but he developed stomach pains, which prompted me to recommend increasing the dose slowly until he tolerated the standard dose. He decided to discontinue Invirase and start another newly approved protease inhibitor called Norvir, but since he was unable to swallow so many large capsules at once, he requested the liquid form, which smelled and tasted like motor oil. At his insistence, he stopped AZT and switched to two recently approved agents in the same class as AZT that could be combined with a protease inhibitor. A month later he complained that Norvir was rotting his teeth, which I thought unlikely in only four weeks. It also disturbed his sleep.

By this time Bruce had exasperated me. "Too bad," I noted in frustration on a pink message slip that was later taped into a progress note on his chart. In such moments it was easy for me to focus on the personality of the man suffering from the disease but forget the disease itself. Terminal illnesses often bring out the worst in people, especially in the denial and anger phases. In this case it brought out the worst in both of us, and I struggled to keep my frustration from getting the better of me. When you're fighting for your life, nothing is really irrational. It's the equivalent of thrashing in the water to keep yourself from drowning. With each telephone call I paused, took a deep breath, and stepped back, repeatedly admonishing myself to be more patient with Bruce. On his request I switched him to yet a third approved protease inhibitor called Crixivan, but after one dose he developed what he described as extreme abdominal pain and gas. I convinced him to resume it, explaining that if he didn't take his medications consistently or properly, he would die.

By mid-July he'd adapted to his three-drug regimen and never missed a dose. I was amazed at the astounding progress he'd made, despite his erratic course of treatment, since his hospitalization in January. He no longer needed a cane because his motor function had returned to near normal, and he could finally live alone without assistance. Unfortunately he lost his clerical job because in his weakened state he took too many breaks. If he'd been employed by a large corporation, he would have been eligible for benefits afforded by the Family Medical Leave Act (FMLA), which was designed to protect people with disabilities in the workplace, but Bruce worked for a small business owner whom the act exempted.

The brain infection, in any case, had altered his personality and impaired his intellect. No longer hostile and combative, he'd become docile and childlike, which further precluded him from holding a job. He became a regular visitor to our office, dropping by on any pretense to say hello, give me a hug, and chat with my staff. Far from being annoying, he was lovable, and my staff always welcomed him. As time passed it was difficult to remember how irritating he'd once been, but the "new" Bruce, zapped of ambition and completely dependent on the social safety net, saddened me. Still, his physical recovery was miraculous, a true medical success story.

Bruce wasn't my only success. Scores of others were having remarkable responses to the new HIV treatment protocol. It was like watching a horror film in reverse: the knife flies out of the body and into the hand of the murderer, the splashes of blood are reabsorbed, the person rises Lazarus-like from his deathbed, flushes again with color, and resumes a normal or near normal life as if nothing momentous had happened. Large lymph nodes disappeared; a mouth and tongue speckled with white patches became pink and shiny again; rashes subsided; KS lesions faded and vanished without a trace; fevers and sweats ceased and pounds lost were regained; smiles returned to faces once creased with anguish and fear.

In the management of HIV infections, 1995 and 1996 were watershed years. By the end of 1996 we had five anti-AIDS drugs in one class (AZT, ddI, ddC, 3TC, d4T), one in a second (Viramune), and three in a third (Invirase, Norvir, and Crixivan). Just three years earlier most of us had despaired of controlling the infection. The word *cure* wasn't even in our vocabularies, and the idea of remission was a fantasy. For several years the Treatment Action Group (TAG), an AIDS activist organization, had published an "Annual Drug Company Report Card" to evaluate the pharmaceutical industry's inadequate response to the AIDS epidemic. Each company received grades for the speed of protocol development and overall drug discovery, responsiveness to community activists, innovation, pricing, and scope of effort. In 1993 most of the companies received Ds and Fs. I did not have an opportunity to view another report card from the group, but once the goal of effective therapies had been achieved TAG remained a gadfly, pressing for sustained research into the long-term effects of anti-HIV medications.

Most remarkably, activists and scientists had come together to pressure Big Pharma and the FDA to speed up clinical trials and pump out medications that promised to rein in HIV. I'd been skeptical about this policy initially, especially in the early days of HIV therapy. But now that scientists had arrived at an effective strategy to combat HIV with three-drug combinations, I was a supporter. Side effects be damned—no side effect was worse than death from AIDS. If 10, 20, or 30 percent of people taking these drugs suffered heart attacks or developed cancer as a result of treatment, that statistic would still pale in comparison to a death rate of 98 percent. Only rabies has a higher fatality rate than untreated HIV. No other infectious disease in human history has had the potential to kill a greater proportion of those exposed to it than HIV. One hundred or even fifty years ago, AIDS might have wiped out much of humanity.

Studies demonstrated that three-drug combinations—two from the first class and one from the second or third class—worked best in bringing the virus under control and preventing the development of resistance, especially in patients who'd never taken any HIV medications. The treatments appeared durable in the majority of people enrolled in trials. After almost a year, the combinations continued to suppress the virus, with improvement in immune system function and a reversal of the downward spiral in health. How long the treatments would work no one knew. People who'd developed resistance because of previous exposure to AZT, for example, alone or in ineffective two-drug combinations, didn't fare as well as the patients who were "naive" to treatment. After a few months those people who were "pretreated" were at great risk of becoming resistant to the third drug too. Somehow Bruce maintained his sensitivity to the various drug combinations, perhaps because early on he never stayed on any medication long enough to develop resistance. Addressing that problem in less fortunate patients with more new drugs was a matter of great urgency, the next frontier in the war.

The results of studies with three-drug combinations were officially broadcast to the world at the International Conference on AIDS held in Vancouver, British Columbia, in July 1996. I was there and the news electrified me. For the first time I paid attention to most of the lectures, because the science of HIV had ceased to be theoretical and could now be applied to my practice. Before that, my mind would go numb and I would fidget and check my watch when a lecturer waxed on about some esoteric aspect of the immune system or a new discovery about the structure of the virus. Now I had the tools to make a good number of my patients better, like a surgeon in the nineteenth century who, after the invention of anesthesia, could operate without strapping down a screaming patient.

Although normally overcast and rainy, Vancouver that exciting week in July was sunny and mild, as if in climatological celebration of what we hoped would be the turning point in the AIDS epidemic. Rejoicing, Gavin and I rode bikes through that picturesque city. We made our way into some of the attractive neighborhoods before entering Stanley Park, pedaling along its scenic lake and shady paths and then proceeding to the city's sandy beaches, where we battled the stiff wind blowing off the Pacific Ocean, our shirts billowing out and flapping like sails. We got as far as the Museum of Anthropology but turned back because it was getting late, forgoing a chance to glimpse Wreck Beach, a gay nude hangout. We left Vancouver on a high note, eager to put our new knowledge to work.

Shortly after their release the various anti-HIV drug combinations were referred to as "cocktails." Images of martini glasses or other containers filled to the brim with colorful capsules and tablets, or hands cupping multicolored pills of different shapes and sizes like rare jewels, began to appear in the press. Some patients were taking dozens of pills a day, when you included treatments to prevent opportunistic infections and vitamin supplements. One of my patients would take a handful, shove them into the back of this throat, and wash them down with a gulp of water without choking, demonstrating the benefits of a well-tempered gag reflex. Later the cocktails acquired a scientific nomenclature, highly active-anti-retroviral therapy, or HAART.

From studies of frozen blood samples stored in research centers around the world during the late 1970s and 1980s, we learned that people with the lowest baseline viral levels (or viral loads) appeared to progress more slowly toward AIDS and death than those with high viral loads. It was determined that, on average, it took ten years from time of infection to the development of AIDS. An uninfected person or one responding well to HAART would have no detectable virus; a person with a raging infection might have very high levels of virus. The curve was bell-shaped, with a minority dying within a year or two of infection or twenty years later. Imagine a train moving from point A to B, where B is AIDS or death. The CD4 count, a reflection of the state of the immune system, tells you how far you are from that destination; the viral load tells you how fast you're moving toward it. The lower the CD4 count, the closer you are to developing full-blown AIDS. The higher the viral load, the faster you'll get there.

Some researchers in 1996 were so enthusiastic about the new therapies that they broached the possibility of a cure. "The next 3–8 months of study data may well answer the question of whether HIV can actually be eradicated in an infected person," Dr. Martin Markowitz of the Aaron Diamond AIDS Research Center in New York said. *Time* magazine named one prominent scientist, Dr. David Ho, its "Man of the Year" for his groundbreaking work in the treatment of HIV, which many people thought would lead the way to that cure.

In Ho's studies of patients treated shortly after they first became infected, the virus couldn't be located in the usual places like the lymph nodes, spinal fluid, gastrointestinal tract, semen, or solid organs. But when he stopped HAART after two or three years of therapy—the amount of time he estimated was required for eliminating HIV, based on HIV's life cycle—the virus suddenly reared its ugly head like a wild beast teased out of the deepest recesses of its lair, to everyone's dismay. It was then that we realized that HIV lay dormant somewhere, hibernating like a bear waiting for the spring thaw. If the winter lasted long enough, the bear might die, but it was later theorized that it could take seventy years or more for the body to rid itself of every last viral particle. Current medications and medications in the pipeline were able to control HIV infection for an indefinite period, perhaps a lifetime, but not eradicate it.

Despite that disappointing discovery, the success of HAART surpassed all expectations because many of us had thought the therapies wouldn't work for more than a couple of years. AZT had failed after a few months. Why wouldn't a three-drug regimen also eventually fail? We were so used to failure and false hope that we disbelieved the evidence around us. The virus remained suppressed and the destruction of the immune system halted as long as the person stuck to his regimen. Like any revolution, none of this happened overnight. The true turning point in the history of the AIDS epidemic in the United States would span another decade, when survival rates far exceeded death rates from AIDS as more people gained access to treatment and an array of medications became available to treat those resistant to earlier therapies.

You'd think that such an achievement would have led to a Nobel Prize in Medicine. But the Nobel Prize is awarded to individuals for their seminal discoveries in various scientific fields and economics or for their work for the advancement of world peace, not to large for-profit corporations like Big Pharma, which often bought promising drugs developed elsewhere and marketed them as their own. Yet what the combined efforts of ongoing research and the pharmaceutical industry had achieved in the treatment of HIV/AIDS was nothing short of astounding. From a universally fatal disease, HIV/AIDS gradually transformed into a chronic one like diabetes. HAART was nearly everything we'd hoped for—and for those of us who had lived through the worst of the AIDS crisis, it was almost beyond belief.

: 14 :

Transitions

(2007–14)

On June 7, 2014, I got married, six days after the state of Illinois legalized same-sex marriage. We headed to Daley Plaza with two other couples and descended to a charmless room where an affable clerk, who didn't bat an eye at six men in suits holding hands, issued our marriage certificates. The setting was hardly romantic, more like visiting a polling place or the Department of Motor Vehicles to renew your driver's license, but for us it was a landmark moment.

In the 1980s the idea of same-sex marriage seemed preposterous to me. I couldn't imagine two men exchanging vows while friends and family cheered them on. What changed my mind was the argument that marriage equality is a human rights issue: same-sex couples deserve to be treated with as much dignity and respect as heterosexual couples. Before passage of the law, you might not have had the right to sit by the side of your ill or dying spouse in a hospital or share in decisions about care; if you died, greedy or insensitive relatives could evict your partner from the home you shared together but to which he might not be legally entitled. The law in Illinois had passed by the slenderest of margins because a lawmaker left an intensive care unit where her son lay gravely ill to cast the decisive vote. It would have insulted her courageous act not to get married.

By 2014 same-sex marriage was largely a formality, the consummation of decades of struggle. The real excitement had come on June 1, 2011, when civil unions for the first time legitimized our relationships in Illinois. In front of television cameras and the national press, we joined sixty other prominent members of the gay community in Millennium Park, the de facto heart of the city, for a grand celebration. It was a glorious day under a blue sky, and the flowers, grass and trees glistened with dew. With Tom and three friends as witnesses, we exchanged vows, kissed, and shed tears, as a lesbian judge we knew sanctified our union. Chicago mayor Rahm Emanuel and Illinois governor Patrick Quinn gave rousing speeches before a jubilant crowd. A handful of people behind a protective fence heckled the proceedings, predicting the end of the world, but everyone ignored them. Some even took selfies with them to commemorate our victory.

At the end of May 2014, only a few days before our marriage, I'd turned sixty years old. For more than thirty years I'd been dealing with HIV/AIDS. So much had changed, and not only in how we managed HIV infection. Although 1984 had looked nothing like George Orwell's dystopia, 2014 looked nothing like 1984, at least in terms of American society's perceptions of the LGBT community. Even the term LGBT (or later LGBTQ) had no resonance in 1984. At that time we belonged to the caste of untouchables. Thirty years later more than half the country supported same-sex marriage. It's not a stretch to claim that without AIDS, same-sex marriage might not have come to pass as soon as it did. By bringing so many well-known, talented, and influential people out of the closet, AIDS paradoxically humanized gays and lesbians. AIDS didn't accomplish this feat alone, but it was an instrumental factor, especially after it ceased to threaten mainstream America and was transformed by the miracle of modern medicine into a chronic and manageable infection.

But I didn't marry Gavin. In 2007 Gavin had split with me after nearly a quarter of a century. The rupture caught me off guard. There'd been no lengthy battles or secret affairs, just the usual disagreements between two people who live together for a long time.

One morning as I was drying off in our water-streaked translucent shower stall like a naked specimen in a museum diorama devoid of props, Gavin made a pronouncement that, like my decision to join Tom in medical practice in 1984, altered the trajectory of my life. He sat on the ledge of the bathtub in a pose that reminded me of August Rodin's famous sculpture *The Thinker*. Our bathroom was capacious, half the size of our bedroom—my mother joked that she could live in it—and glowed in morning light that filtered through a wall of glass block and a large skylight. Moving both hands decisively to his knees, but looking at the marble floor, he announced that he was having dinner with a mutual friend that night. Ordinarily the announcement wouldn't have been a big deal, but the tone of his voice suggested something more ominous.

"Am I invited?" I asked.

"No," he said.

"No? That's really rude," I replied.

After a pause during which several emotions flashed across his face in that soft, diffuse light—sadness, anger, and finally defiance—he said, "I've rented an apartment."

"An apartment?"

"Yes, an apartment. I've leased it for a year and I'm moving out."

The friend he was having dinner with had helped him find it. It was several miles north on the lakefront, not far from his office, in a building that was as ornate as ours was contemporary.

"You should know I've been unhappy for fifteen years," he said.

"Fifteen years?" I said.

I felt my lip twitch upward and eyes squint with incomprehension and confusion. *Who is this person?* I wondered. I stared at him in bewilderment, as if he were a doppelgänger who'd commandeered the body and mind of the man I'd slept beside nearly every night and shared nearly every day of my adult life.

"Wow, that wasn't my experience," I said in a near whisper. "Overall, I've been happy."

Suddenly I grasped that my happiness had been a joyride for one and Gavin's companionship an illusion. I was overcome by an odd sensation, like flying through clouds and seeing nothing but a billowy void while searching for some recognizable object to latch on to and orient me. Although it seemed that I was moving, nothing on my body moved except the water that dripped down my face, arms, torso, and legs. *How could two people have completely different experiences of a relationship?* I asked myself. The answer, which Gavin didn't provide, was too painful for me to contemplate. Instinctively I wrapped a towel around my waist to protect something I never thought needed protection, my soul—or however one characterizes one's persona—as manifested by my naked body. Standing before him in the glass box, I felt ashamed, even ridiculous, in my awkward vulnerability, as if we'd just met and I was being judged, and not favorably.

Mystified, I asked if he'd considered couples counseling. No, but he'd made up his mind after several sessions with his own therapist. I immediately hated his therapist and the friend who colluded with him. I accused him of having an affair with the friend at the encouragement of the therapist, but he shook his head vehemently in denial. He got up without looking at me, refused further discussion, and walked out of the bathroom. I listened to the receding footsteps, click-click-click, on the wood floor in the hallway, then the galloping taps as he descended three flights of stairs and the faint whoosh of a shutting door. That was that—twenty-four years vaporized in five minutes.

A month passed before he moved out, and those were days full of awkwardness. Neither of us knew how to behave toward the other. What conversation passed between us centered on the banalities of life and steered clear of the obvious topic. He might have left sooner had he not suffered a heart attack. The decision to leave me had been more stressful than he let on or I imagined. It struck as he was traveling to visit his sister in southern Illinois. While pausing at a rest stop he developed crushing chest pain, shortness of breath, and drenching sweats and felt nauseated and faint. Frightened, he called me and described his symptoms. Even though I was mad as hell at him, the heart attack shocked me. I urged him to go the hospital immediately, but he decided to go to his sister's home instead.

For two days he languished in bed, too weak to move. After returning to Chicago, he spent a week in the coronary care unit at St. Joe's. Every evening I sat at his bedside as if we were still partners before his discharge to our house, where I hovered over him and hoped that somehow he'd change his mind about leaving me. Three weeks later, after an argument about the future of our relationship, he told me that he felt that he was under my thumb. I didn't understand what he meant; he didn't explain. In anger I replied, "The thumb is lifted. You're free. Now go to your apartment."

A period of darkness followed. Not only did I grieve the loss of Gavin's love, but I also missed his camaraderie. As physicians in the same field, we frequently discussed interesting or difficult cases in our kitchen or bedroom as if attending an informal morning report or Grand Rounds, or vented our frustrations with cranky patients and skanky HMOs. Both our families had embraced us as a couple, and we shared most of our friends. We'd also spent more than twenty years exploring the world together, traveling to six continents and places as remote as Timbuktu and the Komodo Islands — although a late remark that he'd sworn off Third World countries and regions colder than seventy degrees should have alerted me to a deep dissatisfaction. Six months before the breakup, he had exploded in uncharacteristic rage when I chided him for forgetting to book time off for a weekend in the Southwest. The outburst took me aback because he'd never behaved that way toward me before. Three months later, on a trip with eight friends to the south of France to celebrate his fiftieth birthday, he sat as far as possible from me at the communal dining table, rode in a separate car on excursions, and hardly spoke to me. Although we slept in the same bed, he came to bed late, avoided my touch, and turned his back toward me. It was a display of contempt that puzzled me and deeply hurt my feelings. I didn't raise the issue at the time, and I didn't confront him when we returned to Chicago. I wished it away, not recognizing his behavior as another warning sign of profound discontent. How ironic that as doctors we could bring up some of the most difficult subjects imaginable with our patients yet avoid far less monumental ones with each other. The ones that counted in our personal lives were the ones we shrank from for fear of conflict. We both hated conflict.

As I reflected on our relationship, it became clear that tiny seismic disturbances over twenty-four years had created cracks that I never noticed, and the building one day crumbled under the force of its own weight. I wondered when things had begun to fall apart. If it was fifteen years back, as Gavin said, that was 1992, the height of the AIDS epidemic, but also the year one of his brothers died at the age of thirty-eight of lung cancer. Gavin had suffered a number of other losses in the intervening years: Bob, a fellow family practice resident, of AIDS; his closest friend from medical school, C.R., of encephalitis in 2000; his father's wife and then his father; his mother; his oldest sister. These deaths were earth-shattering for him, though as people do, he seemed to recover from each after a suitable period of mourning. I wonder if he had perceived me as distant at those times. I'd like not to think so, but, once again, it wasn't something we discussed. As late as November 2006, when we traveled to Italy with his sister and her husband, he seemed to enjoy my company. We made plans for the future. Never for a moment did I think our relationship wouldn't last a lifetime.

Something changed in the final year. What that was I could never truly know because Gavin became as inscrutable as Bartleby the Scrivener, adamantly refusing to discuss the reasons for the impending breakup. Every time I brought up the subject, he rose as if catapulted by a spring and threatened to leave the room. My mind spun; my jaw clenched; a weight compressed my chest. His reaction to my probing evoked a kaleidoscope of conflicting feelings. I could only speculate on his motives, but speculation is one-sided and one half of a reality.

I asked Tom not to tell anyone about the breakup, but like King Midas's barber, who whispered into a hole inhabited by the mountain god Echo that Midas had an ass's ears, Tom could never keep a secret. Within days, word of our split spread, and I lost control of my narrative. Friends and acquaintances plied me with questions and offered their sympathy. When one remarked, "We all held you both up as a model for the gay community," I felt like a failure, for in my imagination I had held myself up as a model in a microcosm of humanity where relationships rarely lasted long and monogamy seemed the exception rather than the rule.

Thank goodness for my practice, I thought at the time. My patients' illnesses and concerns provided welcome distractions from my own sorrows. I listened to them with greater sympathy and was less inclined to rush to judgment, even if their worries were disproportionate to their symptoms. Yet I found it ironic that after conversing with, examining, and counseling a score or more people each day, fielding dozens of phone calls, and answering an equal number of emails, I'd be overcome by loneliness each night in a house with too many rooms for one person. The telephone there was silent, and the only mail I received was an endless stream of solicitations for charitable contributions and unwanted magazines like *American Cheerleader* and *Boy's Life*, courtesy of the American Academy of Family Physicians, which had sold my name to advertisers. My main solace was a blind and feeble geriatric dog, Fiona, who survived for nine months after the breakup. I had to pick her up to lie next to me in bed, a comforting presence but not a substitute for a lost love. While I grieved and remained immobilized, Gavin moved forward on a new journey from which I was barred.

A painful year passed before a handful of friends encouraged me to move on. For the first time since 1983, I faced two daunting issues: finding another partner and avoiding HIV. Although I'd been immersed in HIV medicine since the beginning of the epidemic, HIV had ceased to be a personal threat after discovering that Art, who'd died twenty-three years earlier, hadn't infected me. Since that time Gavin had been my only sexual partner. The dilemmas confronting my HIV-negative single patients now became my dilemmas. If my patients reflected the gay community at large, 20 percent of gay men in Chicago had HIV/AIDS. Perhaps if a medication had been approved to prevent infection, I'd have been less concerned, but no such medication had yet been proved to be effective in 2008.

I knew you couldn't get HIV from kissing and that condoms worked, but how would I really feel about an HIV-positive partner?

The prospect made me wary, not because I worried about caring for a sick person—that's the usual destiny of one of the partners in a long-term relationship—but because I didn't want HIV. Over the years I'd witnessed a number of different story lines, from abject fear of HIV leading to a life of celibacy to a cavalier disregard of a partner's HIV status. I fell into a gray zone somewhere in the middle but more toward the fear end of the spectrum than the cavalier. Science and irrationality warred within me, and it wasn't clear which might dominate.

Although transmission of HIV from oral sexual contact was uncommon, it wasn't impossible. Sometimes people bleed from the gums or harbor sores like herpes or syphilis, which increase the risk. I also knew that some people lie about their HIV status. Years passed before one of my patients admitted to his lover that he was infected with HIV, and this was only after his lover discovered through a life insurance examination that he himself was HIV positive. When confronted, my patient turned the tables. "You never asked me," he said with a callousness that left both the lover and me momentarily speechless. Others are afraid to disclose their status because they fear that word might spread or that a potential sex partner will reject them. It's hard enough developing intimate relationships; HIV makes it harder.

Barhopping wasn't an option for me. I knew too many people in the Chicago gay community as patients. On the few occasions that I'd gone to Sidetrack, Hydrate, Big Chick's, or Roscoe's with out-of-town friends, the patients I encountered were friendly but guarded. Those on the prowl retreated like lions caught in the act of stalking prey. Others sought medical advice, not certain what else to do or say. In such situations I became self-conscious because I too had to maintain my dignity. Cruising or getting smashed—not things I would usually do—was out of the question. For the same reason—and the fact that I'm slow at embracing new technology—internet hookup sites like Grindr and Scruff or their equivalents at the time didn't interest me.

I turned to the more anodyne websites like Match.com. To my dismay, a good number of matches there also turned out to be my patients. They weren't looking for me specifically or I them, but the site matched us, which I guess isn't surprising. The men I didn't know whom I contacted disappointed me. My salvation was Match. Tom: in 2009, two years after Gavin left, Tom introduced me to Ted, who sat with him on the board of a charitable organization. Although Ted had been a patient of Tom's for a decade, I'd never seen or spoken to him. Socially our worlds overlapped, but somehow our paths had never crossed. At first I didn't want to be introduced to him, since he is fourteen years younger than I. "Oh, he's an old soul," Tom said. "Don't worry about the age difference."

I was wary. But after another Match.com failure—an awkward dinner with a man who looked like an elderly President Nixon and had far less personality—I called Ted and suggested meeting for coffee. If we didn't hit it off, I thought, I could easily escape. Ted insisted on dinner. Reluctantly I reserved a table at a restaurant in a sleek new hotel not far from the long-ago location of Alfie's, where Art and I'd first hooked up. The neighborhood had become gentrified and fashionable, couples pushing baby carriages and women in mink and heels having replaced men in leather chaps or tight-tight jeans.

When I arrived, I surprised a colleague, an infectious disease specialist and another pioneer in the fight against AIDS, who was having a drink with a woman who wasn't his wife. He shifted uncomfortably as we exchanged a few pleasantries. I went to the bar and stared at my cellphone, trying to lower my anxiety level with a glass of wine. Ted had called me to apologize for being late—traffic was heavier than he'd anticipated. He soon walked in at a rapid clip, and we went into the dining room.

Physically, Ted was my type—shorter than I, shaved balding head with a neatly trimmed salt-and-pepper beard, sparkling green eyes, and a warm smile that lit up a handsome face. He wore a sport jacket over a loosely buttoned white shirt with dark chest hairs poking out and spoke in a pleasing tenor voice (he'd studied opera in college). It was a conversation of Wagnerian proportions, lasting six hours, until the weary staff kindly chased us out. A few days later, when a restaurant server we both knew clapped her hands in approval after asking us if we were dating, I realized that I could fall in love again. From that day forward we were inseparable. The news prompted my mother to note that I'd "robbed the nest" and wonder, "What's with you and Irish men?"

By this time my relationship with my mother had shifted from evasiveness to full disclosure. We'd grown closer after my father's death in 2002 at the age of seventy-seven. His death had come unexpectedly, from complications of diverticulitis. Up to that point he'd been in excellent health. Shortly before my father's hospitalization my mother underwent hip replacement, a procedure she'd put off for months despite great pain and difficulty walking. It had been at my father's urging that she finally agreed to have surgery. She bled profusely afterward and was confined to bed for weeks. While she was in the hospital recuperating, he'd spent every day and evening at her bedside. Now she could barely be with him during the greatest crisis of their fifty-two-year marriage. It was heartbreaking when with both hands clutching her cane as she stood at the foot of his hospital bed gazing at his unresponsive body, she whispered a tender farewell.

My mother's emotional dependence on my father had been greater than I'd imagined and exposed a vulnerability I'd not seen before. In reaction to his death, her weight dropped to 80 pounds from 95, and at 4 feet 10 inches she'd lost her dynamism and appeared frail. A gust of wind could have thrown her to the ground, breaking the hip that she'd already broken twice. Her grief lasted a year and a half. After that her voice regained its familiar strength, although she never regained the weight. That vulnerability evoked an instinctive desire to protect her—but she needed no protection and never asked for it.

When I had announced with embarrassment that Gavin and I'd broken up, her posture changed and attention sharpened, much as mine does when a patient reports a symptom that indicates something more serious than a cold or stomach bug. She wasn't surprised, she said, noting that it had been "a good run." It was Mother's Day 2008, and I'd taken her to brunch at an elegant restaurant in Winnetka, a bastion of white heterosexuality. It's not clear to me why I chose that moment to tell her, several months after the fact. Perhaps it was the glass of wine that relaxed me or the charming, homey atmosphere (white tablecloths, subdued natural lighting, profusion of spring floral arrangements, and friendly staff)—or the weariness of a fugitive sick of hiding.

"I never understood why you two were together," she said without missing a beat, indicating that she'd wondered about the nature of my relationship with Gavin for a long time. But seeing my puzzled expression, she added, "But then I never know why any two people are together." She named other unlikely couples in our extended family.

When Ted and I celebrated our civil union in 2011, my mother attended happily. She got along well with Ted's mother, chatting at length with her about who-knows-what, later confiding, "I really like your mother-in-law." She displayed signs of support in smaller ways too, like refusing to eat at Chick-fil-A because of its chief operating officer's antigay remarks and opposition to LGBTQ rights, and sending a birthday card to Ted with an "Equality Forever" stamp on the envelope. She became a true friend. But she always had been a true friend, a fact that had taken decades for me to admit. In the interval I'd expended a lot of energy limiting her to the outskirts of my life, in part because it took me forever not to feel ashamed about being gay.

I reflected on the good relationship I had with my mother during my childhood, before the difficulties of adolescence and beyond. One of my earliest pleasurable memories dates to the age of five, when she turned me into a butterfly for Halloween at my request. She'd sewn wings onto a bodysuit and created a small hat or headband with antennae on it like those on a TV set of that era. Kneeling, she made adjustments holding the pins in her teeth, like the daughter of a tailor that she was or the wardrobe designer that she aspired to but would never be. It was a weird costume for a little boy, but everyone in the neighborhood knew me as the kid with the butterfly net who chased every butterfly he caught sight of. She also helped me with art projects, because I shared a talent for painting and drawing with her, and endured hours of tedious piano practice when I played the same sonata repeatedly until I got it right, even when it drove my three brothers crazy. It was not her idea for me to play the piano. It was something I asked to do, and she gave me her full support. As a child, I did my utmost not to disappoint her. And for the most part I didn't. But it had been that fear of disappointment that prevented me from having a more fulfilling relationship with her from adolescence onward.

Dealing with my mother's death wasn't as difficult as I expected, not because I'd accompanied so many patients on their death marches but because my mother was remarkably brave, clear-headed, and unsentimental about her mortality. During the last six months of her life, she battled a rare form of leukemia. I called to check on her every day, sometimes two or three times. I'd awaken in the middle of the night drenched in sweat, worried about her health. But it turned out that I was more worried than she was. After a bout of severe vertigo that provoked a fall and laceration of her scalp, she joked as I drove her to the hospital, "You prepare for the worst, and when the worst happens you don't know what to do." I think that was true. In fact, the only reason she had told me about the vertigo was that I called her the following morning. It wasn't the first thing she mentioned in our conversation either. She didn't want to bother me, she said when I asked why she hadn't called me after the fall. There were times when she phoned about something trivial, as when she accidentally brought home an orange she forgot to pay for from the grocery store. She didn't want anyone to think that she was shoplifting. But when she had a dangerous fall, not a peep. When offered chemotherapy, she told her doctor with the utmost sincerity not to waste it on her but to give it to young people who needed it more.

My mother died suddenly, one month shy of her eighty-sixth birthday, in November 2013. One afternoon she'd lunched with a relative. The following day she developed pneumonia but refused my offer to take her to the hospital or prescribe antibiotics. The next day she didn't answer the phone despite multiple calls. I knew what this meant and asked Mary, my business manager, to cancel my patients that day. It was a dreadful moment when I unlocked the front door of her house and found her dog Chip, a Maltese the size of a large rabbit, waiting for me in the foyer, tail wagging with uncertainty. She wasn't in the rocking chair or on the couch in the living room, where I'd left her the day before. NPR didn't blast from the radio in the kitchen. The house was eerily silent, the habitat of ghosts, the only sounds my breathing, Chip's panting, and the soft thud of my shoes as I trudged up the carpeted stairs to her bedroom, fearing and knowing what I'd find.

Somehow she had made it up those stairs. It was a peaceful, if surreal, scene. Dressed in her nightgown, she was lying half in bed, half out. Her left index finger supported her chin, and her eyes stared into space. She appeared frozen in time, lost in thought, her face pallid and her lips blue-violet. I phoned Ted, who came within the hour, at which point I broke down. My youngest brother arrived a bit later and had to be coaxed into the bedroom. I phoned my two other brothers in Georgia and Florida, who were shocked and struggled to understand my awkward descriptions of the cause.

I've often thought about how differently my mother's death was handled from that of many of my patients. In the 1980s and 1990s, the partners of my AIDS patients who died at home endured interrogations by a detective, although when the presumptive cause of death was revealed, the detective and paramedics backed off and the coroner badgered me not to demand an autopsy. To the investigator it wouldn't have mattered if the partner had murdered his lover: fear of the disease—or a moral judgment passed on the deceased—trumped all other considerations. On several occasions I didn't give in and refused to sign the death certificate without a definitive diagnosis, especially for a person who was HIV positive and not yet diagnosed with end-stage AIDS, at which time death would have been expected.

I also realized that any number of funeral homes would have accepted my mother's body. More than two decades earlier, funeral homes had been quite wary if the dead person was a single man of a certain age residing in a certain zip code in a certain city. In the late 1980s one funeral director threatened to have my license revoked because I'd failed to inform him beforehand that the person he just embalmed had been an AIDS patient. Had he known, he said, he would have refused the body—a remark that infuriated me. It was, after all, the era of universal precautions, when healthcare workers (morticians included) were expected to adhere to strict guidelines on how to deal with the body fluids of anyone, dead or alive, HIV positive or negative. In deference to the family's request, I'd listed lymphoma as the primary cause of death but omitted AIDS as a secondary cause on the death certificate, which at the time could have become part of the public record. Although I was guilty of omission, I'd assumed that the family had made the director aware of the diagnosis when he accepted the body, but they had not. Nothing I said assuaged him. Fortunately for me, we were on the telephone—otherwise he might have punched me. His complaint to the Department of Professional Regulation triggered a brief inquiry, and for a year I was monitored before the case was dropped. It had been just a minor nuisance.

My parents' decision to forgo funeral services was a relief to me, and my brothers didn't disagree. Having witnessed so many deaths professionally, I dreaded funerals. I understand their necessity, and for those with religious convictions they offer comfort at a time of great sorrow. Some of the services I attended moved me to tears not because I derived any solace from the pastor or rabbi but because I just felt sad for the loss. On such occasions I wished I shared the congregants' faith in God or belief that there is a higher purpose for our existence. But death on an unimaginable scale, sometimes from disease and sometimes in the name of some religious or political ideology—the apparent hallmark of the twentieth century—had wrung any vestige of piety from my soul.

Over the years death has obsessed me, and increasingly as I grow older and continue to ponder the purposelessness of life. We come, make our brief mark on the world, and vanish—that's a cliché but a simple truth. So many lives lost to AIDS, I thought, a surfeit of grief that almost negated my ability to experience grief at all. When someone dear to me dies or I contemplate my own mortality, I often think of the wry yet profound (and depressing) observation in the Portuguese novel *The Year of the Death of Ricardo Reis*. After one dies, a poet tells the novel's protagonist, there is a period when one can roam the earth and put things in order. "The usual period is nine months, the same length of time we spend in our mother's womb," the poet says. "I believe it is a question of symmetry. Before we are born no one can see us, yet they think about us every day; after we are dead they cannot see us any longer and every day they go on forgetting us a little more and, apart from exceptional cases, it takes nine months to achieve total oblivion."

Epilogue

(2016 and Beyond)

In late May 2016, a twenty-four-year-old man named Allen made an appointment to see me for what he thought was an ulcer. When I entered the exam room, I knew at once that he suffered from something more serious. Ringlets of blond hair looped over a bony forehead like branches of trees over a receding shore. The fluorescent light glinted off his brow, cheekbones, and nose and cast his hollowed orbits in shadow. His clothes hung loosely on a thin frame. A wave of dread passed through me, bringing back memories of the old days when young men like Allen sat pensively in my waiting room or languished in the beds of 11 West, now long repurposed.

It had been almost a decade since I'd cared for someone with advanced HIV infection, and I hadn't lost a patient to AIDS since 2004. Once a master of the art of HIV medicine in the era before HAART, I'd almost forgotten how to treat opportunistic infections. Now I would need the internet to guide me. In 2016 most of my patients with HIV were vigorous and healthy, their virus kept in check by powerful medications. The others were afflicted with maladies that had nothing to do with HIV, such as diabetes, heart disease, or an enlarged prostate. Colds were colds and flus were flus, a purple splotch a bruise and not KS. If I saw a yeast infection on the back of someone's throat, it was due to a steroid inhaler to control asthma and not a deficient immune system. If a patient complained of a bad headache, its cause was muscle tension or a migraine, not a weird fungal infection inflaming the meninges, the delicate membrane covering the brain, or a brain swollen by a tumor. I thought of that aphorism from medical school: when you hear hoofbeats, think horses, not zebras: common diagnoses first, oddities last in your differential diagnosis of symptoms. Instead of five to ten per month, perhaps two or three of my patients might die each year, and that would be from diseases that usually kill people, like cancer or coronary artery disease. In thirty years I'd come full circle: except for the fact that the majority of my patients were gay men, I now had a typical primary care practice.

Without voicing a concern—Allen was new to my practice and I didn't want to scare him—I introduced myself and shook his cool hand, then settled onto my stool, opened my laptop, and began to record his story. My fingers were poised over the keyboard, ready to document his words verbatim. I thanked my seventh-grade typing teacher for giving me skills I never knew I'd need fifty years later. With pointed questions I tried to keep Allen on track, because people ramble when talking about their symptoms, giving you information they think is important while you try not to interrupt too often to get the information you need to make a diagnosis. After breaking up with his boyfriend three months earlier, Allen said, he became depressed, stopped eating, and lost ten pounds. But four weeks later he was back in Boys' Town in search of new conquests, the old lover forgotten. Six weeks or so after the breakup, he contracted "food poisoning." His stomach felt on fire and he had severe diarrhea; that lasted just a day, but he had never fully recovered. Since that episode he'd lost more weight, felt bloated, and continued to have bouts of loose, watery bowel movements. A few hours after downing three shots of whiskey one Saturday night in a gay bar, he vomited multiple times. That's when he decided it was time to see a doctor. Friends referred him to me.

Before getting sick, Allen had felt as well as any twenty-four-year-old young man should and weighed 160 pounds. Now he weighed only 139. The last doctor he'd seen was his pediatrician before he left home for college at the age of eighteen. An HIV test performed earlier in the year at Steamworks, a gay bathhouse, had been nega-tive, he said. He'd never contracted any sexually transmitted infec-tions, and he denied topping or bottoming anyone recently, which would have put him at risk for HIV. I doubted his story about safe sexual practices but said nothing. Unless you've known them for a long time, people fudge the truth about their sexual activity. There's a great deal of denial about what really happened in the backroom of a bar or in the dark recesses of the bedroom. Often drugs or alco-hol clouds memories.

I asked him to strip to his underwear and climb onto the gray-leather exam table so that I could perform a thorough examination. He sat awkwardly, shoulders hunched, hands squeezed between his knees, and toes touching the step below. With the exception of his thin appearance, Allen had no hallmarks of advanced AIDS like swollen lymph glands, a yeast infection in the mouth, or purplish lesions. Looking for evidence of CMV in the eyes is difficult with the standard equipment, so I didn't bother to look, but Allen re-ported no loss of vision. Under my stethoscope, whose diaphragm I moved casually across his back from the sharp shoulder blades to the lower edge of his ribs in a zigzag pattern, his lungs sounded clear to me, and he didn't have the characteristic staccato cough of PCP, brought on by the slightest effort at deep inspiration. I asked him to lie down so that I could listen to his heart and then gently press on his abdomen in search of an enlarged liver or spleen. With each breath I could observe the expansion and contraction of the individual ribs of his ribcage because of the loss of body fat.

Since the recent HIV test had been negative, I suspected that he might be suffering from the symptoms of newly acquired HIV, not AIDS. The timing seemed right. As early as two weeks after being ex-posed to HIV the virus runs wild, invading every organ in the body, before the immune system responds and in most people negoti-ates a tentative truce that only one side honors. During that spree—known as acute retroviral syndrome—the infected person often, but not always, experiences symptoms like fever, drenching sweats, persistent cough, diarrhea, weight loss, and extreme fatigue. He can look like someone with advanced AIDS. The syndrome sometimes last for months, like a case of mononucleosis. You don't see it often, even if you're an AIDS specialist, and it's easy to miss because it can mimic a dozen other illnesses. Further complicating a diagnosis of acute retroviral syndrome, HIV may be one of several sexually transmitted diseases, like syphilis, gonorrhea, chlamydia, herpes, and hepatitis or an intestinal parasite like giardia, imparted simultaneously during a single fateful sexual encounter. I would have to check for these problems in addition to screening him for HIV.

After getting dressed, Allen admitted that he didn't always practice safe sex. As we spoke more about the risk of HIV infection during unprotected sex, he grew visibly alarmed. He wanted to discuss "PrEP," or preexposure prophylaxis, which involved taking a medication that the Food and Drug Administration had approved in 2012 and the Centers for Disease Control and Prevention promoted to prevent HIV infection in people at risk of contracting the virus. If taken as directed, that medication is more than 90 percent effective in preventing HIV infection, almost as good as a birth control pill to prevent pregnancy. I explained to him that before I could prescribe PrEP, I had to be absolutely sure that he wasn't HIV positive. If he was, he might become resistant to that medication, which would make future treatment more difficult.

I sent Allen's blood sample to an outside lab. If negative, the result would be reported in twenty-four hours. If positive, it would take several days more because of further testing to confirm the diagnosis. I imagined that the wait would create intense anxiety, disturbing his sleep with anxious half-dreams and distracting him during the day from his work as he contemplated the implications of a positive diagnosis. I recalled the unbearable two-week wait for the results of my own HIV test thirty years earlier. When you fantasize about winning the lottery, you think about all the wonderful ways you'll spend your money—the new house, world travel, meaningful donations to needy causes. When you're waiting for the results of an HIV test, you think of the worst scenarios—the difficulty of finding a partner who won't be afraid to touch you; coming out of a different kind of closet; an early death. The knowledge that they've been infected with HIV devastates most people and fills them with an aching loneliness that few others can feel or comprehend because HIV infection has so many more ramifications than other life-threatening illnesses, like cancer, or ones that can kill you quickly, like the Ebola virus. I still can't really comprehend it, even after witnessing hundreds of deaths from it and caring for more than a thousand men harboring it.

Allen was one of twenty patients that day. Many of the others were also interested in or already on PrEP. In recent years, that has become typical. I spend a lot of time counseling single men or men in "open relationships" about how to protect themselves against HIV. In an open relationship, men with partners or husbands don't hide the fact that they're having sex with other men. In the age of PrEP, fewer men use condoms, and barebacking—that is, men fucking without condoms—has resumed where it left off, as if the nightmare years of the 1980s and 1990s had never happened.

I wholly endorse PrEP, just as I wholly endorse oral contraception for birth control. I don't buy the argument that the birth control pill or PrEP encourages promiscuity. Men, and gay men in particular, are promiscuous, have always been promiscuous, and always will be if given the opportunity. The treatment and prevention of HIV infection is a public health emergency and will continue to be a public health emergency until we have a cure or an effective vaccine to prevent infection, neither of which is on the immediate horizon. HAART and PrEP are our best bets for eradicating the AIDS virus. If everyone infected with HIV took HAART and every person at high risk of HIV infection took PrEP, the epidemic could end in a generation. But denying the reality of human sexual behavior fuels epidemics rather than extinguishes them. Thirty-five million deaths from AIDS and another forty million living with HIV today are the price the world has paid for such denial in the early years of the epidemic.

But PrEP doesn't prevent other STIs. Every week I see someone with rectal gonorrhea or chlamydia, and every few months another case of syphilis. Before AIDS, sexually transmitted diseases in gay men were almost as common as colds. But as in the aftermath of a hurricane or other natural disaster, once a community has been rebuilt, life returns to a semblance of normal. Before PrEP and the decline of condoms, many of my patients would almost certainly have acquired HIV, of that I'm convinced.

Unfortunately, Allen's HIV test was positive. He'd also contracted syphilis and giardia, which gave him three reasons to be ill. I phoned to let him know the results, and he agreed to come to the office the following day to discuss what to do next. When we met, I didn't chastise him for being careless or ask him why he hadn't consistently used condoms or thought about PrEP earlier; those remarks would have been pointless. Instead I gave him a comforting hug.

Then, as I sat facing Allen in the examination room where I'd seen thousands of patients over thirty years, I had fleeting glimpses of the men who'd died before I could offer lifesaving regimens. There was Donald, whose entire arm KS had turned into a bloated, blistered, and useless appendage, the pain so agonizing that only amputation at the shoulder joint provided some relief; and then after dealing with the ghost pains and the loss of his dominant arm, he succumbed to another opportunistic infection a few months later. There was the haunting image of Raoul, who leaped naked from his hospital bed and ran down the hall of 11 West crying out for help in a last burst of energy before dropping dead at the foot of the nurses' station. And there was Philippe, a concert pianist with a brilliant future who flew to Moscow for a piano competition with an IV line that pumped medication to treat a sight-threatening infection, which was then detached for a few hours while he gave the final performance of his life. I recalled my friends and colleagues Neal, Stan, Bob, Ron, and so many others whose stories I'd recorded in my journals and who perished in a war that seemed without end. That was a hell I never wished to revisit. In the waning years of my career, ensuring that none of my patients dies of an AIDS-related problem, or acquires HIV, has become my primary mission.

I thought of the relatively small number of men in my practice who were lucky enough to have survived into the era of HAART. As a result of our early anti-HIV therapy, the majority of them developed lipodystrophy, a strange syndrome characterized by an abnormal redistribution of body fat that often leaves the face bony, arms and legs pencil-thin and roped with prominent veins, and flattened buttocks. Some people acquire "buffalo humps," collections of fat at the base of the neck that can be as large as a softball; "man-boobs," as one of my patients refers to his pendulous breasts; and bellies as rotund as those of a woman in the third trimester of pregnancy. At its worst, the face can look monstrously distorted as if it were embedded in a pillow of fat, and the body shaped like Humpty Dumpty. Yet otherwise most of the people who've developed lipodystrophy appear to be healthy. They're full of energy, have normal appetites, and remain actively engaged in the world.

These strange and sometimes devastating side effects occurred primarily as a result of two medications, AZT and D4T, for reasons that aren't entirely clear. And in these cases lipodystrophy is for life. Over the years plastic surgeons have become more adept at improving the architecture of the face with artificial fillers or fat transfers, but there's nothing that can be done about plumping up the rest of the body or shaving off significant amounts of fat. For many, lipodystrophy amounts to a scarlet letter, a constant reminder of HIV, and for some it is a badge of shame in the outside world. As one of my patients remarked with self-deprecating humor, "Once I turned heads. Now I turn stomachs." Most of my patients have learned to live with it. They're grateful to have survived—AZT and D4T saved their lives—but it's the kind of side effect I wouldn't wish on my worst enemy. Every time I see them, I feel like a surgeon who bungled an operation; I feel responsible for the outcome. But of course AZT and D4T were at one time among the few tools I had at my disposal.

I thought of another group of men who were prepared to die and elected to go on social security disability in the early 1990s, when there was no hope for survival. Inadvertently, HAART created a lost generation, like those who suffered from posttraumatic stress disorder after World War I or II or the Vietnam War and were never rehabilitated to a normal life. Cruelly referred to as GODs, for gays-on-disability, these HIV-positive men waited for the call of the executioner, but the executioner never summoned them. In subsequent years they've been unable to maintain their skills and have scrambled to find a purpose for their lives, with varying success. Most are victims of an imperfect social safety net—if they returned to work, they'd lose their Medicare coverage and access to lifesaving medications; if they remained on Medicare and social security disability, they weren't allowed to work more than twenty hours per week. Unless they had saved vast sums of money, came from a wealthy family, had a boyfriend or husband with a good job, or were lucky to have private disability insurance, they eke out a meager existence on monthly social security checks alone.

When I fill out their disability forms today—a ritual I undergo once a year for each of these men—I'm stretching the truth to a certain degree. Yes, most of them can lift, squat, push, pull, climb, and sit; they can carry on a conversation and endorse checks. By the criteria on the forms, the majority aren't physically disabled or cognitively impaired, but no one would hire them, and they're incapable of holding a job. They're the walking wounded, their impairment no less real or legitimate than that of the traumatized soldier who witnessed the deaths of comrades or escaped his own death by the skin of his teeth.

I still have a good number of long-term survivors in my practice. Many of them will live to be eighty or more. My oldest patient with HIV is almost ninety. Until a couple of years ago, he walked the five miles from his apartment to my office for his appointments. Except for lipodystrophy, you'd never know that he'd once nearly died of AIDS. In the 1980s and 1990s, my go-to consultants were Dr. R. the lung specialist, Dr. F. the retinal specialist, and Dr. A. the gastroenterologist, each assessing various opportunistic infections. Since that time, as my patients grow old, my go-to consultant remains a gastroenterologist, who now performs colonoscopies to screen for precancerous colon polyps, as he does in my HIV-negative patients, but also I call on a urologist, to deal with the annoyances of enlarging prostates and the diagnosis and treatment of prostate cancer, and a cardiologist to manage coronary artery disease or treat heart attacks. Locked away as if in a maximum-security prison, HIV no longer threatens almost everyone in my practice.

"We want our patients to die of little old men's diseases, not AIDS," a friend of mine, an infectious disease specialist, once quipped. And for the most part we've been successful. For those with access to care and who are compliant with their medications, death from HIV is no longer inevitable or even likely.

"Although your virus might not be detectable after treatment," I said to Allen as my thoughts and words returned to his particular predicament, "you will not be in remission, like a person whose cancer has been successfully treated. I hope that won't always be true, that there will be a cure, but I have to advise you based on what we're doing in 2016. You have to be prepared to be on some sort of treatment for the rest of your life. The responsibility for ensuring that you never go without medication will fall on you and on you alone."

I didn't tell Allen that I won't be at his side during those later years to cheer him on, as I had been with the fortunate survivors of AIDS in my practice, because he will outlive me. Maybe no physician will be at his side to age with him, manage his HIV infection, and treat medical problems that have nothing to do with HIV, for fewer doctors are choosing to pursue a career in primary care because of the low pay compared to the income of specialists, and of those even fewer have the expertise or desire to treat patients with HIV. Infectious disease doctors are not trained or prepared to act like primary care physicians; most of what they do is hospital-based. And private practice, in which a young doctor opens an office and spends a lifetime serving a community like Tom and I did, is going the way of the dodo, replaced by physicians employed by hospitals and other organizations. Those doctors, with expectations different from my own, may be less inclined to practice with that sort of dedication and commitment.

Allen listened attentively as I explained how easy it was these days to treat HIV. Just a single tablet, I said, when twenty years earlier you had to take a shitload of medications. You don't have to take it exactly the same time every day, but you need to take it. I don't care if you're vomiting or suffering from depression: don't miss that pill! I assured him that he wouldn't develop lipodystrophy.

After starting his medication, I wanted to see him in four weeks to make sure that his viral load had dropped to a very low level. After that, for the first year he would need to be monitored quarterly, to verify that he was responding fully to his HIV medication and check for early signs of significant side effects; thereafter he would see me twice yearly, because treating HIV for the long haul is, in a way, still a grand experiment. We had twenty years of history with HAART, but not fifty. Perhaps there would be adverse reactions we'd not yet anticipated, or maybe not. He would need to tell his sexual partners about his HIV infection before having sex with them and would still need to wear condoms, or have them wear condoms, if he topped or bottomed with any of those partners, to minimize the risk of acquiring other STIs. The risk of transmitting HIV would be virtually zero if he didn't interrupt his treatment. He could live a normal life, travel anywhere in the world, eat whatever he liked, within reason, and make plans for the future like any young man his age. He nodded in acquiescence.

Allen made it easier for me by not falling to pieces. Throughout the conversation his face remained unperturbed, as if we were talking about something less momentous, like the weather. Perhaps it was the arrogance of youth. At twenty-four, the idea of one's mortality hardly registers. The internal struggle I'd imagined for him as he waited for his diagnosis apparently had never happened—I had been projecting. In the 1980s we had trembled with terror because friends and acquaintances were dying as if randomly picked off one by one before our eyes. In the twenty-first century young people don't know anyone who has died from AIDS, so they're less afraid. Taking just one pill—"one pill, that doesn't seem right to me," one of my long-standing HIV infected patients once said with befuddled amusement—now makes AIDS seem manageable, hardly dangerous at all, like Charles Manson rendered harmless by his lifetime prison sentence.

Introspective and bright, Allen appeared to have come to terms with the possibility that he had HIV in the few days before this visit, and he accepted the results and my upbeat message with surprising equanimity. He was determined to do whatever he could to maintain his health. Once his three ailments were treated, he would regain the weight he'd lost and feel healthy again. Twenty-five years earlier he might not have been so composed and I wouldn't have been so hopeful. After sending his prescriptions to his pharmacy electronically—it still seemed like magic to me—I closed the lid of my computer and we both stood up.

"Thank you for your time, doctor," Allen said without the trace of a tear. "I know I'm going to be OK because I'm in good hands. I promise to be a good patient."

"Yes, Allen, you'll be OK," I said. "But don't do it for me. Do it for you. I can prescribe the medication, but you're the one who has to take it. Now it's up to you."

"Yes, of course."

"See you in four weeks," I said.

"See you in four weeks."

I looked him in the eye and smiled reassuringly. Then I gave him a pat on the back and moved on to the next patient with laptop in hand. Paper charts and scribbled notes were now things of the past, like the hundreds of men I'd lost to the worst disease I ever encountered during my long career. *If I never see another patient with full-blown AIDS again*, I thought as I pushed open the door of the adjacent room, *I'll have absolutely no regrets.*

Acknowledgments

This book has had many iterations from its inception several years ago to its final version. One early reader whom I must thank is Joan Stephenson, who knew at once that the book should be a memoir. At first I didn't know what it was; Joan suggested that I take a class on memoir writing and found Story Studio, a writer's workshop in the Ravenswood neighborhood of Chicago. I was lucky enough to be accepted into a course titled Memoir in a Year, whose instructor, Nadine Kenney Johnstone, was a wonderful mentor and guide. She and my fellow students in the class, Angela Cameli, Ruth Hoberman, William Mansfield, Beverly Offen, Elizabeth Savage, Maria Springer, and Abby Terrell, held my feet to the fire and helped shape this memoir.

Others along the way who pushed me in the right direction were Carlos Mock, Joel Gallant, David Blatt, John Davidson, Sean Strub, Owen Keehnen, and, of course, my business partner—and second husband, as I jokingly call him—Tom Klein, who has traveled unflinchingly with me on this journey for the last thirty-five years. He made many helpful remarks as I wrote and rewrote the book umpteen times. My business manager and dearest friend of more than twenty-five years, Mary Ammons, also gave me some keen advice when she read the book at various stages. But more important, without her loving and clearheaded stewardship of our at times chaotic and heartbreaking practice, I couldn't have survived.

I'd like to give special thanks to Robert Sharoff, who was not only a steadfast cheerleader but a patient counselor during the difficult process of finding a publisher. He was not my agent (I had none), but was better than an agent. Moreover, I'm grateful to my editor, Tim Mennel, for sharpening my prose and forcing me to look deeper into myself when my instinct was to shy away from the more difficult questions.

And last but not least, I must thank my most trusted confidant, loving companion, and insightful critic, my husband Ted Grady. When he pronounced my first tentative steps at writing this book "nitty"—that is, too clinical and not sufficiently emotional—I was surprised. But he was right. I had my work cut out for me.